The Forbidden Body

Shelley Bovey is a journalist and broadcaster specialising in women's issues. Her interest in the topics of women, weight and food stems from a lifetime of repeated dieting, experiencing persecution for being fat and being stereotyped as a large, comfortable Earth Mother. She no longer diets and lives peacefully in Somerset surrounded by large, curvaceous hills and happy, fat sheep and cows. She has a lot of cats, a husband and three grown-up children.

The
Forbidden
Body

Why being
fat is not a sin

SHELLEY BOVEY

Pandora
An Imprint of HarperCollinsPublishers

Pandora
An Imprint of HarperCollins*Publishers*
77—85 Fulham Palace Road
Hammersmith, London W6 8JB

First published by Pandora Press in 1989 as *Being Fat is not a Sin*
Reprinted in 1991
This fully revised, updated and expanded edition published 1994
1 3 5 7 9 10 8 6 4 2

Shelley Bovey asserts the moral right to
be identified as the author of this work.

A CIP catalogue record for this book
is available from the British Library

ISBN 0 04 440871 4

Phototypeset by Harper Phototypesetters Limited,
Northampton, England
Printed in Great Britain by
HarperCollinsManufacturing Glasgow

*To the memory of my parents
And of my dearest friend, Jackie Marcus,
who died as I was finishing this book.*

*For my family
Alistair, Jane, Lindsay and Alex
and for Marion Davidson with love.*

Contents

Preface and Acknowledgements

This book is for everyone. If you are not fat, you will know someone who is. If you don't know someone who is, you will read about being fat, see programmes about it on television, participate in discussions about it. Weight is the one issue about which *everyone* has an opinion. I believe that opinion should be formed by the objective research that has been done in the field — and from the subjective feelings and experiences of fat women themselves.

The first edition of this book was published as a feminist title, but I have since learnt that fat is not a feminist issue. In itself it is not about the inequality of the sexes, although fat women are more victimised than fat men because our society is still not sexually equal. Sadly though, other women are very often fat women's worst enemies. Whoever sets the standard of thinness as the ideal, it is women who rush to attain it at whatever cost and who often denigrate or patronise those of us who do not 'belong' in this way. If only women would realise how much time they spend talking about their weight and what they should or should not be eating, and if only they could realise how boring it is and how destructive of any real female interaction. At a gathering of interesting women writers the other day, someone brought in tea and a plate of cake. The thinnest, most glamorous woman there broke the rhythm of the discussion when the plate reached her. 'Oh no, I shouldn't,' she said. 'I'm *desperately* trying to lose some weight.' This, of course, called forth the Pavlovian response to such a comment: 'Oh no, you *can't be*. You're so beautifully slim . . .' and they were off.

A word about the new title. This book was originally called *Being Fat is not a Sin*, a strong, *factual* statement, and it is still what this book is about. But many women are not ready to reclaim the word 'fat'. To stand in a bookshop in front of a strange sales assistant and ask for that title was too much for some. It meant drawing attention to their size and naming it, using the F-word in the process! What was worse was that I, the author, was beginning to find that the title stuck in my throat whenever I was asked what my book was called. Fat activists will not approve of my evasive behaviour and I apologise to them, but being fat is so painful, such a sensitive issue for so many that I believe we must keep that in mind at all times. I chose *The Forbidden Body* because that is exactly what the state of being fat *is* in the eyes of society, and because the title does not immediately give away the exact meaning of the book. It is also slightly mysterious, which will, I hope, make women (and men) of whatever size pick it up, whereas the previous title left nothing to the imagination and may therefore have been ignored by those who believed it did not apply to them.

One small technical point. Because of my own ambivalent feelings about the word 'fat' I have found it difficult to find an adjective that I am happy with. So I have fluctuated between fat, large, big, overweight without being really satisfied with any of them. I do not believe we have the right word in our language. Similarly, where I use inverted commas to describe size, such as 'normal' weight it means that this is not *my* opinion of what is normal, but that which is imposed upon us.

Since writing the first edition of this book, I have received a wide variety of responses and reactions. Most precious are the letters from women who have said how much it has helped them — in many cases, how it has put into words years of bottled-up feelings of anger, pain and injustice that they have not dared to give voice to, so great is the hatred of fat women and so potent the punishment that society metes out to us. It has been effective in silencing women for centuries but never has it been so vicious as now, in the late part of the 20th century. Many feel so damaged after a lifetime of persecution and assault that it is less painful to protect those raw wounds by meekly colluding with the oppressors than to expose them by speaking out and fighting back. We need every tool available to enable us to do this, and this new edition of my book shows, I hope, that we need never feel alone. There are a great many of us who are ready to work hard to topple our culture's thin-worshipping and there are now more resources to help us to do it.

I have been called upon at times to justify the writing of this book. Many people do not believe that it is in *any* way acceptable to be fat and they consider me irresponsible. They are firmly entrenched in the belief that fat is bad, whether they try to justify this on health grounds or aesthetic judgements. The more I hear this, the more I realise that this — and other books of a similar nature — are urgently needed. Vivian Mayer, who writes under the name 'Aldebaran' is an American feminist and fat activist who began the Los Angeles Fat Underground movement in the early 1970s. Amongst other achievements, these women produced a book of Fat Women's Writings, called *Shadow on a Tightrope*. At the end of the foreword in the edition I have (1983), Vivian Mayer writes: 'I pray for an outpouring of fat women's thought, speech and action, to come soon, in our days.'

An outpouring is indeed what we need. It does not have

to be in books or articles, though these will all help. Women's voices need to be heard, even on a one-to-one basis. Apart from the fat hatred there are also misconceptions, and lack of knowledge and understanding, and while fat women remain silent these things will be perpetuated. Other reactions I have had are: 'Is it really as bad as you make out? Surely this discrimination, this persecution can't be as terrible or as rife as you say it is.' Or they make assumptions: 'You've written this book so you are obviously proud of being fat.' These are the people willing to enter into a dialogue, to rethink their preconceptions and their misunderstandings. They, at least, are open-minded. But whether they are or not — and it is a bonus if they are — we *must* keep saying how it is for us with all the honesty and courage we can muster. So much misunderstanding comes from our silence: 'I never realised you *minded*' is a remark many fat women will recognise all too well. And because I believe we are beginning to establish footholds, it is more important than ever that we do not make a public apology for our size in the form of dieting.

A surprising number of people have written or spoken to me admitting their own, previously unconscious, prejudice. These are the liberal, tolerant, often radical types — the ones who campaign for other oppressed groups, the ones who would never have believed that they could have in any way been oppressors themselves. Reading the book has uncovered their deeply hidden prejudice and it has shocked and horrified them. I am so grateful and moved that they have had the integrity and courage, not just to bring it out and deal with it themselves, but to apologise and admit to it. These people, the champions of human-rights causes, demonstrate how deep the fat prejudice is, how ingrained in the psyche of Western man and woman, laid down at an age before we begin questioning the way the world works, and therefore absorbed into the unconscious.

The overtly prejudiced will continue to pour out their vitriol as long as there is no legislation to curb them, but who knows what changes in their thinking we can effect by refusing to remain passive any longer? There is no individual, no incident, no corporate institution not worth challenging. Even bigots can change.

I have roundly condemned the medical profession for their biased and unsympathetic treatment of their fat patients but to my amazement I did not receive one letter criticising the health sections of this book. Instead a number of doctors wrote and apologised. They explained that they were taught in medical school to be tough with overweight patients, or they simply admitted that they had been prejudiced and unaware of the psychological and physical harm they might have done. I would like to thank them wholeheartedly and hope that they will pass the message on to their colleagues.

I want to do everything I can to stop the persecution, the hatred, the rejection and the contempt directed at fat women. And I want everyone who reads or hears about this book, or about fat persecution, to do or say something, however small. There is a Chinese proverb — 'Even a journey of a thousand miles begins with a single step.' I think we've covered more than a few steps, but we must *keep walking*.

I would like to thank so many people. Firstly, the women — and a few men — who wrote to me after publication of the first edition and who were so affirming. They made me feel that the long, hard graft had been worth it many times over. Getting letters from strangers is such a privilege — they feel like new friends.

Thanks go to Gill Riggs, Pamela Bacon and Carol Carnall who acted as my unofficial press-cuttings service, between them keeping me up to date with reports and features in a variety of newspapers and magazines.

I have made wonderful connections with people internationally who are either working for, or supporting the
cause: Sally E. Smith and everyone at NAAFA; Linda
Omichinski who runs the HUGS programme in Canada;
Mary Evans Young of *Dietbreakers* who has been a good
friend and a constant support; Deborah Vietor-Engländer
from Germany who saw to it that the book was translated
and published over there. I want to thank them for their
input and their friendship.

I must thank the journalists and broadcasters who, with
few exceptions were open-minded and very sensitive in the
way they handled this subject. Being fat is the perennial
cartoonist's delight but only in one or two cases did I meet
with that reaction. The fact that they were in the minority
makes those journalists stand out as vastly inferior to their
professional counterparts.

When researching the medical and health aspects of
weight and dieting I received tremendous help from Andy
Kent and Bridget Dolan of St. George's Medical School,
London. I would like to thank them for taking the time out
of their busy lives to help me with information, research and
discussion. They were both uncompromisingly supportive
and non-judgemental and any woman who receives therapy
from them is lucky indeed.

Although I have not yet met any of the American experts
working in this field, I have had access to their books and
papers which have been invaluable and I feel I know them
already. Thank you, too, to Karl Niedershuh who has given
many years of tireless work to NAAFA and who shared
with me his own personal and painful experiences.

I note that in the acknowledgements to the first edition
I described Marion Davidson as indispensable. She still is
and I re-iterate my thanks for her endless support, her
wisdom and her affection. She has listened for many hours
to me carrying on about What It Means To Be Fat and she

has offered much that has been helpful in the way of insight.

Special thanks for Karen Holden who has been an inspiring and quite wonderful editor with much to bear!

And to my family who know how much they contribute to my life and to my work — at least, I hope they do.

Finally, I would like to thank all my friends, for being themselves, and for being there for me. I most want to thank Jackie Marcus whose belief in me was unwavering and whose friendship was one of life's greatest gifts.

Somerset
December 1993

1

Cut down to size

Being fat is about knowing it. It is about a round-the-clock awareness that the fat person's body overflows the strict boundaries imposed on it by Western social and cultural norms. To be a fat woman means to carry a double burden, for women are expected to conform to a more rigorous and stereo-typed aesthetic ideal than are men. There is no way to hide being fat except by staying indoors, and so most fat women exist within a tense and stressful straitjacket, unable to be freely themselves, circumscribed by social censure, aware every day in everthing they do that they are being defined by their body size. It is only on the telephone that a fat woman can claim equality.

Racism, sexism and ageism have been recognised for the evils they are and brought into the daylight and named. They are part of a process whereby society rejects those who are different from the sociological role model which has been defined as acceptable. Fattism is still largely a *hidden* prejudice and as such it is perhaps the most vicious of all. It is insidious because, couched in concern for the fat person's health and wellbeing, the real truth of blatant discrimination often remains concealed. Fat is hated and despised and fat people are coerced to the outer limits of mainstream society — that is if they dare to try to be a part of it.

Being fat is not about wanting to fit the fashions only

available for the thin, nor is it about wanting to conform in order to be seen as sexually attractive, though both these factors play a part. Being fat is about experiencing hatred and contempt. It is not confined to the young, and it extends beyond the stages where peer pressure is thought to be important. It is about being ostracised and isolated and it can affect any woman who is heavier than the so-called norm. I received this letter from a woman of seventy-five:

I am fat, grossly fat. Each night when I go to bed I hope I shall die in the night. I have tried all diets and calorie counting but I still put on weight. The medical profession has been very unhelpful, indeed criminally so. I seem to be written off entirely and feel of no account whatsoever. As a result of my bulk I cannot take much exercise, have swollen ankles, varicose veins, acute piles, huge belly, huge bottom. Most people I meet are contemptuous and imagine I indulge in an orgy of food. Far from it. Life is bleak and there seems no escape.
I feel so guilty about being fat.
I feel so helpless because I cannot solve the problem.
I feel alone because I am so repulsive.
I feel unwell most of the time.
I hesitate about giving or accepting invitations and try to hide away.
I feel somewhat bitter and resentful of my family's dislike of me. They don't mean to be critical but obviously they are afraid they might grow like me.
How I envy thin people, they look pleasant and have lots of energy.

When I read this letter I was overwhelmed with anger on behalf of this woman. To be fat at any age is painful. To suffer the kind of self-hatred caused by the condemnation of those who should be the most supportive — family and medical advisers — is a searing and diminishing experience. To endure all of that at the age of seventy-five is monstrous.

Later, when I spoke to Margaret Meredith, who wrote that letter, I found a woman damaged but without self-pity. She is *angry* that society wields such power in its judgements and that the individual who wants to fight back is so puny in comparison. In addition she faces age discrimination and with the double burden feels that 'they' would like her out of the way. She refuses to go under though, and in her late seventies and six stone (84lb) overweight, she begs a few questions about the medical Jeremiahs' predictions of reduced life expectancy for the over-weight.

We all need to feel that we belong in the society in which we live. When people decide not to conform it is a conscious choice, a protest of some kind. Anorexia nervosa may be a sickness but it begins with a deliberate choice — to lose weight. No one chooses to be fat. There have always been rebels in society, but very often rebellion takes the form of moving away from the establishment and into opposing, but unified, groups with their own codes and mores. Fat people only group together in slimming clubs.

In the United States, journalist Leslie Lampert wore a 'fat suit' for a week and reported her experiences in an article in the May 1993 issue of *Ladies Home Journal*. Her experience taught her that 'society not only hates fat people, it feels entitled to participate in a prejudice that at many levels parallels racism and religious bigotry ... it seems we are more tolerant of ill-mannered, indecent individuals who are slim than we are of honorable, oversize citizens'.

There is a great deal of evidence (see ch.7) that concern about fat woman's health is justified. But it is misdirected.

Hatred, discrimination and prejudice all considerably affect physical, emotional and mental health. Stress causes high blood pressure. The vilification against fat has got to stop.[1]

Every day the fat woman dies a series of small deaths. It is simply not possible to forget that you are fat when the daily round is an obstacle course of reminders.

A DAY IN THE LIFE OF A FAT WOMAN

Seven a.m. and she gets up feeling tired. She always feels tired, no matter how much sleep she gets. She wonders whether she is lacking in vitamins or some vital nutrient, whether she is working too hard and just not getting enough rest and relaxation. But those rules apply to normal people. *They* say she is tired because she is fat and they do not look beyond that. Her doctor declines to investigate or advise but just gives her a diet sheet which she is supposed to believe is a cure-all for any ills she might suffer.

Washed and dressed, she pokes about in the larder, wondering whether to save calories by missing breakfast. Deciding against it — the weakness and hunger are not worth it in the long run, she eats a bowl of muesli with plain yogurt and leaves the house for work.

Getting into her car for the short drive to the station, she feels that small lurch of apprehension that comes with every journey she does in her car. She cannot do up her seatbelt without it digging in so that she can't breathe out and the top part of the belt nestles right round her throat. Stopping suddenly could strangle her so she drives her car unbelted, breaking the law and feeling precarious and unsafe. She arrives at the station without mishap.

Her train is an Inter-City and always crowded. She makes her way down the central aisle looking for a seat, the focus of many eyes as the train lurches on its way and the cause of irritation to the passengers whose arms she accidentally jogs as she passes them. There are a few window seats spare and she stops at one, politely asking the passenger sitting in the aisle seat to excuse her. He stands up, rather than move over — she doesn't blame him as there is a solid arm rest between the seats and very little space between that and the table. Not easy to negotiate even for the thin and agile. She is hotly conscious of the fact that there is a traffic jam as more passengers try to pass down the aisle looking for seats. They cannot get past until she squeezes into the window seat and the other passenger sits down again. She takes a breath and pulls in as much of herself as she can, then pushes her body into the seat, jammed for a few agonising moments as her stomach sticks on the hard rim of the table and she is wedged astride the central divider. One ungainly heave and she collapses somewhat haphazardly onto the seat. Halfway to London she longs for a cup of coffee but cannot bring herself to go through the seat/table/aisle performance again, so meekly she waits until the train pulls into the station.

She joins the rush-hour throng going down into the underground, where there are turnstiles to be negotiated. People slip through quickly and easily, hell bent on getting to work on time. She squeezes her bulk through slowly, apologetically, again holding people up. The tube is packed and she strap-hangs for three stations. Then seats become available and she sits down, trying not to take up more than her share of space, trying not to overhang the edge of the seat, pulling her legs tightly together so that they take up less room. The woman next to her glares and pointedly moves inwards to the side of the train, taking up less than half the space of the seat.

Out in the fresh air she walks briskly to her office. On the way she walks past workmen on some scaffolding. She tries to shut her ears to their calls, to hurry on, but she hears their jeering tones and just catches the words 'fat cow'.

Her colleagues greet her pleasantly as she walks into the office and hangs up her coat. She is popular at work because she is funny and jolly and never seems to mind when they tease her about her size. In fact, she makes jokes at her own expense. 'Do you think that chair will stand my weight?' she asks, laughing. The women in her office are all slim, but they all believe they need to lose weight. The conversation often turns to diets, aerobics, fasting. 'God, I've put on weight' they will say, pinching the flesh on thirty-six inch hips. Only they don't call it flesh, they call it 'flab' or 'revolting fat'. Sometimes they ask her curiously, as though she were a different species: 'Wouldn't you like to be slim? Have you ever tried losing weight? It must be so difficult to get clothes.' In a strange way, though, they don't include her in their talk of diets, almost as though she is so big she must be beyond or outside the discussions that preoccupy them. Nor do they refer to her when they talk about hair, make-up, fashion. She is not considered a part of these things.

Coffee break and someone suggests they 'sin' by getting doughnuts from the deli down the road. 'Shall we be wicked?' says their boss, a trim woman in her early forties. 'Well, I've been good all week,' says one size ten. 'I'm going to indulge.' She works at her desk, ignoring the arrival of the cakes, wanting one yet knowing it would be perceived as greed.

At lunchtime she has to join her boss and another colleague in a lunch for a client at a smart nearby restaurant. The menu is delicious, but the other three women are making self-righteous noises about salad. They order steak, fish — she looks longingly at the salmon *en croûte* then orders a mixed salad. The waitress approaches with the pudding menu. 'Not for me,' says the client. 'I'm on a diet.' The others follow her example and light up cigarettes as they order coffee. She hates cigarette smoke and longs to be daring enough to order a chocolate mousse. But she doesn't. She dare not draw their attention to her — she knows from experience that the only way to avoid gratuitous remarks about her weight is to give the impression that she is making some kind of reparation for her sin, not compounding it by eating 'fattening' and 'forbidden' foods.

She doesn't return to the office in the afternoon — she has to go to the hospital for a chest X-ray. On arrival there she is asked some routine questions by a nurse who tells her that she is storing up trouble for herself unless she loses weight, and would she like to see the dietitian? She declines. She knows about diets and she knows they do not work — not in the long term.

She is shown to a cubicle and told to undress and put on the gown she will find hanging up. The gown will not go round her and she waits, near to tears in the cubicle, ashamed to walk out half-naked. She tries the gown back to front — that way her breasts are covered but she knows there is an ignominious expanse of bottom showing. She chooses that as the lesser of two evils and is chided for wearing the gown the wrong way round. 'Still,' says the radiographer brusquely, 'With someone your size there's not a lot we can do about the gown.' The chest X-ray involves pressing as hard as she can up against a metal plate. Her breasts are squashed and bruised. After an interminable wait it is over and she can go.

She feels very despondent after the hospital experience and decides to spend the rest of the afternoon browsing round the shops. She is looking at a rail of dresses in a department store when an assistant approaches her. 'I'm afraid we've got nothing in *your* size,' she is told, disdainfully. Retorts rise up and hover on her lips. She wants to point out that she can see for herself what sizes they come in, and that she feels that if they haven't got her size they should be doing something about it. But she hears herself saying apologetically, cravenly: 'Oh no, it's not for me. I'm looking for a dress for my daughter.'

She realises that she needs to get something for supper so she heads for a supermarket. She relaxes a little, walking round the store, enjoying the sights and smells about her. She buys some chocolate biscuits — a treat for the children. She hasn't spent much time with them lately — the working mother's guilt — and she starts filling her basket with compensatory goodies. She looks up and sees two slim women staring at her, their expressions as eloquent as if they had spoken: 'No wonder she's so fat if that's the kind of thing she eats.' Again she feels the need to placate, to apologise for her crime, to choose fruit and salads, visible proof that she is 'doing something' about her anti-social state. For the children's sake she resists the urge to put the chocolate goodies back on the shelves and hurries her purchases through the checkout, quickly hiding them in the store's plastic bags.

She walks to the tube station, braced against the scramble, the squash, the elbow, painful in her breast as someone pushes past. She holds herself tense throughout the journey and all through the tussle at the main-line station. The train is so full she is too weary to struggle down the aisle with the extra burden of her supermarket carrier bag; too weary to squeeze and stumble for a seat, too tense to run the gauntlet of the disapproving looks, the grudging moving aside to let her past, to let her in to a seat for which she has paid like everyone else. She stands in the space between carriages, holding onto a rail, swaying with the motion of the train. Tired again. Is it her fault, she wonders. Is it just being fat that brings about this utter dreariness of body and spirit? And tomorrow will be the same, and tomorrow and tomorrow . . .

Most fat women will readily identify with some, if not all of that imaginary day. It is not an exaggerated account —

all those instances will be familiar and indeed it is perfectly possible that they may all occur on the same day.

Alice Fowler, a British journalist, became a fat woman for a day, and by doing so provided both a subjective and objective insight into the way size really does affect the way the world treats us — *excludes* us. She borrowed the fat-suit used by Goldie Hawn, who, in the film *Death Becomes Her*, is seen to put on a vast amount of weight. Complete with a latex mask, giving her a fat face, Alice Fowler ventured into the outside world:

'Three hours is all it takes to become socially unacceptable,' she writes. 'I don't smell, I'm not drunk, I don't commit a crime; all I do is don a huge fat-suit, adding ten stone to my normally size 10 frame.' Out in a busy street, she found that 'while the world makes way for a thin young woman, it closes ranks against one much larger. Ironically for one so big, I'm almost invisible: a looming shape observed from afar and ignored at close quarters.' In the course of the day, Alice Fowler visits a gym, and while the staff are 'kindly and welcoming', clients using the equipment 'gape in undisguised horror'. It is at this point that Alice Fowler loses sight of her own reality — that she is a slim, acceptable woman. She says: 'I am transfixed by the hostility I sense coming from the other side of the glass. I feel ugly and almost scared. "I can't go in there," I bark, and bolt for the reception area. *I have become the person that I appear to be* (my italics). In my fat suit I find my personality changes. I am grumpy, resentful; as people's attitudes to me change, so mine change to the world around me. I feel closed off, no longer a member of society; as my size has grown my sense of belonging has shrunk.'

Those who believe that fat people are oversensitive, or that they exaggerate the hostility and alienating attitudes of the thin world will surely think again if they consider that Alice Fowler felt as she did after only three hours of living as a fat woman and that she could re-enter the 'normal' world in seconds. The feedback — both verbal and non-verbal — that a fat woman receives when she tries to take her place in a lifestyle enjoyed by the socially acceptable, is very often far too negative, punitive and painful for any but the very confident to ignore.

This is especially true of physical activities. Take cycling — I love cycling but find it an ordeal to ride around the district where I live. 'Mind the wheels don't buckle,' some wag will yell, thinking he is being terribly funny and original. There is no reason on earth why a fat woman should not ride a bike and do so well, but conditioning is such that it is perceived as a joke, a cartoon, and people see what they think they are going to see, instead of power, stamina and elegance.

More than ever before we are exhorted to exercise, to work out, to 'go for the burn'. Running has replaced jogging in popularity and marathons are to be found everywhere. A friend of mine, a large man, overweight — fat, in fact — entered for a fun run in his local town. He was encouraged by his friends and cheered on by the crowd.

In contrast, a woman friend, weighing over 20 stones (280lb) who had nursed a long cherished ambition to run the annual London Marathon could only bring herself to start her training jogs by going out early in the morning, complete with dog and handbag so that if she should chance to meet anyone she could pretend she was just walking the dog. She laughed at herself, we laughed with her, but why should she have had to do it that way? Because she is vulnerable and human and would not risk the jeers and pointing fingers had she been seen in a track suit, openly running. [2]

People imagine that fat women do not take part in marathons because they could not run. They can train to be as fit as anyone but most do not because there is an almost universal fear of revealing their bodies in movement or scantily clad in any way. They are closeted.

The 1980s produced a counter-movement to fat oppression, usually known as Big is Beautiful. This only further isolates fat people, making them another category by the use of positive discrimination. It is the apologists' approach. Big is Beautiful does not attack the worm at the core of the apple; it does not tackle the shadow aspect of fat issues, revealing the dark side of humanity, the side that seems to have a compulsion to victimise, to oppress, to stamp out. Big is Beautiful puts a forced smile on the face of fat without revealing the depths of unhappiness and humiliation that most fat women experience. It is this that needs to be brought out into the open. It has to be recognised. And it has to be stopped.

2

Persecution, discrimination and other every day horrors

After a long period of stress, overwork and general run-down-ness combined with the dreary post-Christmas part of winter, I was given a present by a friend. It was a day at London's beauty and health spa in Covent Garden, The Sanctuary, which offers relaxing and therapeutic treatments as well as the usual Body Beautiful treatments. I looked forward to deep, soothing massage and the jacuzzi in particular. On arrival, I was handed a wrapped polythene package containing two white towels and a white towelling robe. The robe's edges did not even reach my nipples — there was no way I could wear it. On asking for a large one I was told that they were all the same size. They used to have larger ones, I was told, but now just the one — small — size. There was nothing they could do, they said — they were sorry. I had a choice — to walk out and abandon my day or to stick it out somehow. I stripped off my underwear and put my dress back on. The Sanctuary has a beautiful sculpted setting — white, Spanish-style arches, tropical greenery and pools full of exotic fish. There were slim white-robed figures relaxing on couches round the water. I felt hot, red and conspicuous as I moved among them in my dress. I had the massage and the jacuzzi but I did not enjoy the day. Feeling so totally out of place made it impossible.

The next day I wrote a letter to the manager of The Sanctuary, expressing distress on behalf of all fat women and describing the day I had had, while praising the facilities available for women there. I concluded the letter:

> I spent the day in my dress. You can imagine how that spoilt the enjoyment — not only was I hot and uncomfortable but I was the recipient of many stares, never a pleasant experience.
>
> This means that The Sanctuary is only open to women who conform to a certain size, thus precluding many people who, I know, would like to spend a day there. Presumably the only answer for people like us is to fork out and buy our own white robes? I don't think that is good enough, however, and I shall be recording the experience in my book, due out this year, and in a magazine article about The Sanctuary.
>
> I would be interested to hear your comments.
> Yours etc.

I received no reply to my letter which tells me several things: that The Sanctuary had no intention of changing their policy of one-size robes; that they did not feel my complaint merited the courtesy of a reply; and perhaps most important of all, that, to them, fat women were of so little importance that inclusion of this incident in a book and a magazine article was not enough to worry them about bad publicity or about their image. As a journalist of many years experience I have learnt that the thought of adverse publicity terrifies most commercial concerns into at least investigating complaints levelled against them. I would conclude from The Sanctuary's silence that a criticism of their lack of helpfulness to fat women would count as no criticism at all. It seems like another instance of the powerlessness of the oppressed.

I was given a further insight the next day into the strength of the hatred felt towards fat people. The friend who had given me the present was recounting the incident with some heat to a colleague. Her colleague's response was equally heated. 'They only have small robes,' she told my friend, 'because a place like that is not meant for fat women. It's really offensive to have to look at women like that — it must have been awful for everyone else there. She (me) should not have gone there.'

Brutal, vitriolic, fascist even. Yet that woman was only being honest. She was stating what is largely felt by society, though most don't have the courage or perhaps the insensitivity to lay their prejudices out in the open with such frankness.

My friend asked her colleague why she was so violently opposed to the idea of a fat woman in a health spa. 'Fat people are revolting, disgusting,' she was told. 'People paying a lot of money to have a relaxing day at a health place should not have to cope with such a grotesque spectacle. They smell. They are lazy and they take up too much room. Fat people should pay double fare on public transport.' There was a good deal more in the same vein. I asked my friend where she thought her colleague had acquired her violent feelings of antipathy. She replied that this particular woman prided herself on her slim figure and on the effort she put in to maintain this. The effort consisted of self-control where eating is concerned and self-discipline in the form of exercise. Together, these two virtues amounted to self-respect. This one woman, whose outburst was prompted by the thought of me, a fat woman, despoiling a place meant for the Beautiful People, encapsulated the attitude of our society in a single voice.

In Oakland, California, newspapers published letters from people complaining about fat women jogging around Lake Merritt.

NAAFA Newsletter, October 1989

FAT IS DIFFERENT

Prejudice towards and hatred for fat people is a double edged oppression. However deeply racist, sexist, ageist or anti-semitic some people may feel, they are encouraged in Western society to quash those feelings, and for obvious good reasons. It may amount to tokenism but the civilised level of communal behaviour is that those who differ in colour or religion should be integrated, albeit uneasily, into white Protestant Western society. After all, people can't help having black skins, can they? So runs the thinking of the nominally racially tolerant. But fat? That's something different, because fat people *can* help it. They don't have to parade the results of their gluttony, their abandon, their over-indulgence, lack of self-control, lack of self-respect, their overflowing, visible, tangible evidence of immoderate behaviour. They should do something about it. It is this condemnation, alongside the hatred of the fat itself that makes society's alienation of the overweight more concentratedly powerful than that of any other minority group. But as American researcher, Dr Paul Ernsberger points out, to expect a fat person to become thin is as unreasonable as expecting a black person to bleach her skin or a Jew to convert to Christianity.[1]

A man was taken off a South West Air plane by four armed policemen because he was 'encroaching' on his neighbour. And Sally Smith, Executive Director of NAAFA, has to buy two seats when she flies, though no airline in America will grant her double frequent-flying miles. It is not uncommon for a large passenger to have to buy two seats.

The Times, 20 April 1992

To be fat means never to be able to conceal the thing which society hates. A smoker without a cigarette, an alcoholic without a drink can choose not to arouse hostility. A Roman Catholic or a Plymouth Brother looks like anyone else. And though blacks, like fat people, cannot hide, they also cannot do anything about their skin, nor do they touch the centre in another person which says 'Ugh. I could so easily become like you'.

Any good psychologist will tell you that condemning other people for no good reason is a reliable indication that the person who condemns is unhappy and insecure. Contented people do not need to hit out at others, savagely and gratuitously. The worst kind, in my opinion, are those who have a public platform — usually in the media — and who use their inner fear, confusion or hatred to ridicule or revile others. The effect of this is to attract followers who get some sort of vicarious satisfaction, rather like the voyeurs who gather ghoulishly at the scene of a road accident. It is the dark part of human nature operating, the side that wants to witness violence. As fat-baiting has had no restraints of any kind imposed upon it, anti-fat viciousness has no boundaries.

Consider Lynda Lee-Potter, right-wing tabloid journalist, commenting on a television series in which the character played by one of Britain's best actresses, Judi Dench, was deserted by her husband. She deserved it, says Lee-Potter, because she was 'so overweight, unkempt and bovine'. In response to angry readers' letters, Lee-Potter wrote that

> Letters from outraged fatties have poured in . . . The main message is that the overweight are constantly upset at being pressured by the media. But since there are so many portly bodies around, I can only suggest they're not pressured enough. However, I shall bravely continue to do my worst.[2]

And she did. In an article which began:

> There have been some daft organisations over the years, but the National Association to Advance Fat Acceptance must be one of the most silliest and most damaging.

she attacks a simple statement by Executive Director, Sally E. Smith, that 'Women are starting to realise that their size is not their fault.' This obviously pushes some buttons for Lee-Potter who rants about it being 'fatties who control their intake of doughnuts, éclairs, Mars Bars, hamburgers and suet dumplings' and who don't have much fun 'running through the surf in a swimsuit if you're so hefty you look as though you could kick-start Concorde'. The lady seems afraid of Fat Acceptance; she says 'The new cult will no doubt be adopted over here, so I'd like to deliver my own blow against spreading thighs — in aid of common sense.' But instead of following with her definition of common sense in this context she goes on to say that it is not a commodity often seen in American women and then continues to insult both fat women and Americans. Another clue comes at the end of the piece, when she writes about 'an increasing cult which tells people they should love themselves as nature intended', but then changes from the general to the specific, thus revealing her own uncertainties about herself: 'But personally I feel that nature is unfairly selective, unjust, with a nasty streak of malevolence, and that it's up to most of us to fight her every inch of the way.' Speak for yourself, is the retort that springs to mind — but that's just it — she is. The final clue comes in her claim that 'Middle-age should be the time to have the chance to be selfish and self-obsessed.' These are two of the negative qualities ascribed to fat people by those who hate them, yet described by this woman as 'pleasures'.[3]

Sometimes the 'fat-bashing' is meant to be humorous.

Like the YOU Magazine (*Mail on Sunday* Colour Supplement) Journo-lists: 'Do you have a weight problem? Ten telltale signs' . . . of which some are: 'Your private health insurance company suggests a group rate; you dream of being as thin as Roseanne; the local Scouts use your old raincoat as a marquee . . .' and so on. Or 'Dr Beach's guide to seaside etiquette' by John Diamond (supposedly a serious journalist) in *SHE* (supposedly a serious magazine, concerned with important issues). He gives 'advice' to made-up agony-aunt type letters about the way women supposedly feel about lying on the beach. 'On every beach' he says to one 'correspondent', 'there's at least one other beach bum built like Roseanne Barr's fat sister. Go lie next to them. And every time you feel like pulling your waist in . . . you must look over to the barrage balloon lying next to you on the sand and ask her whether she would like to borrow a guy-rope to tether herself down with. You would be amazed at just how much thinner that makes you feel.'[4]

I don't think this so-called humour needs any comment from me. The authors of this sort of thing are the losers, not those they target. It's too silly even to come under the heading of persecution. But unrestrained prejudice or ridicule can rarely be so dismissed because it is a sword that pierces to the core of an already fragile being. When this book was first published in October 1989, I found myself 'viciously lampooned in print' as one journalist described it. I received a call from Val Hennessy of the *Daily Mail* in which she said she would like to write a piece on the book and suggested she took me for lunch at the Savoy, one of London's most prestigious hotels. We met and went into the dining room. 'I hope you're going to eat a nice big lunch,' said Hennessy, which alerted me to what she might be trying to do — although I had no idea of the extent of her merciless intentions. I decided that I would behave totally naturally and not try and give any impression at all, just be my usual self. We looked at the menu — 'Go on, have that — and that — and that,' said Hennessy. I told her I loved fish and we ordered salmon with sturgeon eggs as a first course, followed by poached brill with lobster mousse and ravioli. As we ate, Hennessy constantly urged me to have more, to have second helpings, bread rolls, more wine. I would have done if I had wanted to, but the truth was that the two fish courses were utterly delicious and very filling. 'Now pudding' said Hennessy, and even when I said I was full, she insisted the waiter bring the trolley. I'm not a great sweet eater and I really didn't want anything. I did not have a pudding and I remained calm throughout the interview, though by now I had a fair idea of what was going to happen.

What happened was a full-page article in the *Daily Mail*. Hennessy quotes herself as saying: 'They've got some lovely salads on the menu . . .' and follows this with: 'whereupon Bovey, bosom heaving, specs steaming over, bellows: "How dare you assume I want a salad . . . Why the hell should I deprive myself?" And it's clear she isn't going to deprive herself this lunchtime as she butters herself another roll and drools over the hors d'oeuvre trolley. *Tartare de saumon* with sturgeon eggs arrives, and she roars "They've forgotten my eggs. I want my eggs", until a frazzled waiter replaces it . . . Bovey laughs, great self-deprecating chuckles that make the cutlery vibrate and the dessert trolley rattle.' In between Hennessy's vile and made-up pen portrait of me, there are her versions — with varying degrees of accuracy — of what I wrote about. When the second course arrived, she reports: "Yum, yum, are there any vegetables?" shouts Bovey. "And some potatoes please and a drop more wine." She tucks in.' Then comes the final, most despicable lie. Hennessy wasn't going to let my refusal of pudding interfere with her caricature — she just made it up: 'Round comes the dessert trolley. Bovey chooses chocolate profiteroles and cream. "Good on you, Bovey, let it all hang out," I start to say, but she's banging the table and ranting through a mouthful of profiteroles . . .'[5]

When I first read this article, I was devastated. Although I'd been a journalist for years, I'd obviously retained some sort of naiveté — or is it just that you think it can never happen to you? Whichever it was, I couldn't belive it *had* been done. What had I done to this woman that she could write something like this? In time, I realised that this was a perfect example of tabloid journalism. She probably thought it was a clever way to write about a woman who had written a book defending fat people. But most of all I saw the clearest evidence I could possibly have had — because it was personal and first-hand and *public* — that persecution, oppression and humiliation are a vivid reality, that we are the target of a no-holds-barred, unrestrained and unqualified victimisation. I believe Val Hennessy wrote that piece because that is how she sees fat people as a whole and she did not let her disappointment at my normal behaviour stop her from inventing what she failed to experience or see in me.

It is a psychological truth that we react most strongly against those traits in others that we suspect we may possess ourselves — and do not want to own. The thin hate the fat because if they relaxed their own rigid control they just might find they are capable of overflowing their tightly set boundaries. Hilde Bruch, a psychiatrist and one of the pioneers in the field of the psychology of weight, remarked that she had often observed real envy in the constantly dieting, thin-obsessed parents of fat children — because the child was 'daring to satisfy the same impulses which the parents keep under strict control. It seems to me that something of this order is expressed in the public's hatred of people who do not control their impulses to eat and so become fat'. And Llewellyn Louderback, author of

Fat Power (a marvellous and liberating book) points out that 'those who force themselves to go without find it absolutely intolerable that there are people who, in their view, refuse to "exercise self control"'.[6] Natalie Allon states that it is the middle-class white woman who wants to lose 25-40 lb herself who censures the overweight woman, even while she berates herself.[7]

A New York Assemblyman once suggested that since obesity is the result of 'an addiction for food', all cases should be uniformly reported under the city's drug addiction laws.

From *Fat Power* by Llewellyn Louderback

In a lifetime of being fat, I have observed that it is those who fear putting on weight who treat my size with the most aggression. I spent a miserable year working with a radio producer who spent her time fighting her own natural and extremely pretty curves. It took a third party to point out to me why I was at the receiving end of so much hostility. Every time she sees you, she is made aware of what she could become, I was told. And indeed it proved to be so; in a rare moment of mateyness during a studio editing session, the producer offered me a confidence: 'It takes will-power and self-control,' she said patronisingly. 'Look at me. You wouldn't believe it, but if I weren't careful all the time I could soon end up looking like you'. This was borne out by several of the women who wrote to me with their feelings and experiences for this book — it was those with a minor degree of overweight who were the most critical of other fat women:

'I'm size 14 and I should be 12. I am lumpy, full of ugly bulges, unfit and *very* unhappy about it'. Interestingly, this woman went on to refer to fat women as 'them' rather than the 'us' used by most correspondents:

> I think *all* fat people are undesirable. Fashion passes them by for obvious reasons; I don't think people pay much attention to what they say, do, write or achieve generally, no matter how gifted they are. Deep down most people dislike fat people and act accordingly.

There is truth in this woman's last sentence. The dislike comes from low self-esteem and is externalised in the sort of oppression and persecution I have begun to describe in this chapter. In *Overcoming Fear of Fat*, a collection of essays, the editors, Laura Brown and Esther Rothblum identify fat oppression as 'a catalyst for energy-draining self-hatred'. This self-hatred is internalised in the form of a desire to lose weight — surveys have shown that *whatever they weigh*, nearly every woman would like to lose at least 7 lb — and externalised as a projection onto other women — condemnation through fear. I believe these factors influence the writing of Lynda Lee-Potter, Val Hennessy and others like them — especially when they keep returning to the subject, as Lee-Potter does.

There is another kind of fat-oppressor: the woman who has lost control of her life and uses dieting as a focus for regaining control over *something*. Nina Myskow, who was a television critic for a tabloid newspaper, decided to diet at the age of 40 and weighing 11½ stone (160 lb). Before then her eating was wildly out of control. She had, she says in her autobiography[8], 'all the control of a perished panty-girdle'. In the book, Myskow catalogues a round of sex, parties, drink and shopping. She is frequently 'completely smashed', and says she has always spent more than she has earned and has had her cheque book and credit cards removed by her bank. Then she went on a much-publicised diet and lost 2½ stone (35 lb), and became an unashamed fat-hater:

I think letting yourself be fat and wearing drab tents and support sandals is a negation of sexuality . . . Besides — I fancy men who fancy thinner women, I don't fancy men who fancy elephantine sixteen-stone women who look like their grannies.

Her fear of fat was such that she couldn't bear Weight Watchers because 'they were obsessed with elephants and I'm sorry, I don't want to identify with people who are six stone (84 lb) overweight'.

We live in a time of excesses and of chaos and when women's lives seem to mirror this, they grab onto the one thing they can control — their weight. Nina Myskow says 'My life is a total fuck-up' and this statement is the cornerstone for her obsessive weight control. Acceptance of 'elephantine' women might lead her to relax her own rigid hold on her diet — so her defence is scorn, ridicule and of course, prejudice.

We went to shopping centers, amusement parks, places where there were many children. We had a brief consent form saying that we needed photographs of children for a study and asked every parent who passed by to let us photograph their children. No parent of a thin child ever refused consent. No parent of a fat child ever gave consent. Sometimes parents permitted their thin child to be photographed, while hiding their fat child behind them.

Wayne Wooley, Ph.D of the University of Cincinnati
Eating Disorders Clinic

I am often asked why I think fat prejudice is so very strong and so venomous. I think the answer is best expressed by the wise Australian psychologist, Dorothy Rowe: 'To go beyond fear we have to accept ourselves and to let other people be themselves and to accept them as they are.'[9] This can help us to understand why fat people are so hated and I hope will enable those who feel almost paralysed by a life-time of persecution to take one small step towards a sense of self-worth by understanding that the bully is more fearful than the coward. Those that oppress us have not learned to accept themselves.

Prejudice is something that children learn at an early age. Studies have been done in America in which children were presented with six black and white line drawings. These depicted a 'normal' child, a child with crutches and a brace on one leg, a child in a wheelchair with a blanket covering both legs, a child with one hand missing, a child with a facial disfigurement and a fat child. Subjects were asked to assess the pictures in order of likeability. The results were almost always unanimous. The 'normal' child was preferred. The fat child was the least liked.[10] It is not difficult to understand how easily young children learn that fat is nasty and to be avoided. It is a subject that is discussed with tedious monotony and regularity. So a small child may carry in her mind the image of her mother, looking in a mirror and saying half to herself: 'Oh dear, I'm putting on weight. Don't want to get like Mrs so-and-so.' And conversations between adults so often contain versions of 'Have you seen X? *Hasn't* she put on weight?' In this way a small child will very quickly perceive the negative attributes of this thing called weight, and by the time she starts school she is already primed to abhor this condition in her peers and in their mothers. What she has learned at home will be fuelled and fed by the remarks and jeers she hears other children make, either about a fat child or a mother. My son said to me when he was very little and had been at school a couple of terms: '*Why* aren't you like the other mothers?' I was sad for him and for myself and I could do no more than to bring up my children to look for people's qualities instead of evaluating them by their appearance. But I realise what tremendous peer-group pressure I am trying to counteract. It is at this early stage that I think schools could and should play a much more active part in shaping young minds, and who knows how things might change if fat-baiting were caught at birth, as it were? However, it is deeply rooted in our culture to congratulate people when they lose weight and while that happens children will continue to absorb the idea that fat equals bad.

Recent years have shown significant changes in children's literature. Awareness of our multi-cultural society, of different sexual orientations, of age and of disability has been reflected in many of the excellent children's books of the '80s and '90s. Even in our television-dominated world, children are exposed to books and influenced by them. Yet because there are no laws, written or unwritten, to prohibit fat-bashing, one author at least has found an easy platform on which to ridicule fat. The book is called *Mrs Circumference* by Catherine Storr.[11] The story is in rhyme, starting with a description of the eponymous lady: 'As fat as a pig? Three times as big . . . she was as large as a hot air balloon.' It goes on to say that if she travelled on public transport, Mrs C took up too much room, 'More than she oughter', so that people said 'that a lady so large had no call to be on Public Transport at all'. Catherine Storr is insidious in the way she communicates her message; in places you can almost imagine her whispering behind her hand to an engrossed child: 'So when she went for her daily toddle — (I could say a waddle — But wouldn't that be too unkind?).' She catalogues the lady's eating habits and her inability to buy clothes to fit: 'She couldn't buy dresses. Wherever she went — She had to make do with a small bell tent.' One day she gets on the underground in London — the Circle Line — and cannot get off. So what happens? She goes round and round for so long that she has nothing to eat and of course she *loses weight*.

Catherine Storr misses no chance to moralise 'To be such a size is not only sad — It's also incontrovertibly bad,' and she also sows the seed into young minds for a future eating disorder: 'Will she have learnt the lesson that — Missing meals can make you less fat?'

WOMEN AND HOLY MEN

Hatred of fat, as an outward and visible form of self-indulgence, is often stated as being based upon the Protestant ethic of ascetic impulse control and the virtues of self-denial.[12] This Puritan ethic also reinforced abhorrence of two of the seven deadly sins, gluttony and sloth and throughout history fatness has carried a label of sin and immorality. There is a mediaeval painting entitled 'The Last Judgement' by Lochner which encapsulates this unequivocally. The sinners, who are being dragged off to Hell, are all fat, while the blessed ones bound for Paradise

---

What I see as a cultural historian of dieting is a society fearing that it is out of control, equating leanness and fiber with predictability, regularity and moral strength. A society unsure of its own rewards and confused about the nature of its sustenance, where it calls excellent meals 'almost sinful'. This is a society in which feeling fit has become a spiritual category, where fitness means . . . you are morally just. This is a society in which fat represents not only unfitness, but spiritual backsliding, or an utter failure.

Hillel Schwartz, author of *Never Satisfied:*
a Cultural History of Dieting, Fantasies and Fat

are all slender. A lesser-known aspect of the seven deadly sins is that in England in the 13th century, Archbishop Peckham ordered every priest to preach on the sins four times a year, and to add 'branches' to each of the seven and preach on them as well. It was thought that each of the principal sins would lead on to secondary ones; thus pride produced ambition, vainglory, boasting, hypocrisy, etc. With gluttony, there was 'mental dullness, excessive talking, buffoonery, and uncleanness of any kind' — an incongruous association but characteristics still attributed to fat people today. Certainly this morality was strongly reinforced in the middle ages but it did not begin there. It is necessary to go right back to the dawning of Christianity, to the early Fathers of the Church, Tertullian, Augustine and Jerome and to their interpretation of the words of Christ himself, in order to find the tap-root of this two thousand year old hatred and fear of flesh.

Where fear is greatest, condemnation will be the most harsh, the most damaging and ultimately the most destructive kind. What the early Fathers feared most was women. Women were the object of classic psychological projections by these holy men who so feared their own sexuality that they invested women with powerful lusts with which they inflamed helpless men; even the angels were not able to withstand '. . . virgins, whose bloom pleads an excuse for human lust . . .'.[13] If angels were not proof against the sexual lures of women, drastic measures were called for.

Priests were constantly being reminded of what happened to Adam. In a letter from St Jerome to a young priest[14] we read the following: 'Remember always that a woman drove the tiller of Paradise from the garden that had been given him'. The letter goes on to say that should he (the priest) fall ill and need nursing, he should make sure he received the ministrations of a mother or sister. If a relative were not available, the Church maintained many elderly women for such a purpose. Jerome continues: 'Never sit alone without witnesses with a woman in a quiet place.' With such power to corrupt as was invested in women, it is easy to see whence spring the roots of misogyny.

Woman, we are told, is man's deepest enemy. She is the harlot who will lure a man to his doom because she is Eve, the eternal temptress.[15] It is taken for granted that she is overflowing with lust. It comes as no surprise to learn that St Jerome was 'one of the greatest voyeurs of all time'.[16] He is rampantly frustrated, so he tells women that *they* are rampantly frustrated, and he tells women that *they* are sexually insatiable. And if a woman dresses attractively, she is crying out for sex: 'Her whole body reveals incontinence.' Thomas Aquinas believed that woman was 'defective and misbegotten, for the active force in the male seed tends to the production of a perfect likeness in the masculine sex, while the production of woman comes from a defect in the active force . . .'.[17] Even Aristotle came to the conclusion that the biological norm is the male. Every woman is a failed man.[18]

It was not enough, in the early Church, to be a virgin — a woman also had to make herself as sexually repulsive as possible. And certain early Roman women, wanting then as now to please men, embarked on a life of asceticism and mutilation, removing as far as possible any traces of womanhood, both physically and spiritually. Thus the 'transvestite saints', women who, believing the Church's teaching that sanctity was only achieved by being male, cropped their hair and fasted their bodies into a state of androgyny. They wore male clothing and often took the masculine version of their name; some even entered monasteries. They were not looked upon as oddities, not ridiculed nor reviled. They were canonised. The earliest feminists?

We should not overlook the power that the early church had over the development of so-called civilisation. Christianity was powerful, influential and political. So when we talk about its effect on women, we cannot confine this effect to a few dotty saints. The teachings of Augustine, Tertullian, Jerome and Aquinas stand up today as pillars of philosophical thought. They were great men in many respects and if their wisdom is still respected in some areas, it is not surprising that their paranoia and hatred of women have descended down the ages still causing ripples.

A *Ladies Home Journal* survey found that American women were twice as afraid of getting fat than of 'all the hate and killing in the world'.

From *Fat Power* by Llewellyn Louderback

Food and sex were always inseparable in the minds of these men. And while women with their sexuality were dangerous, then the answer was denial of all sensuous pleasures, of anything in fact that fed the flesh rather than the spirit. Fasting brought about chastity and therefore sanctity. Jerome wrote: 'Not that God, the Lord and Creator of the universe takes any delight in the rumbling of our intestines or the emptiness of our stomach, but because this is the only way of preserving chastity.'[19] Flesh satisfied with food will rise up against the soul and precipitate the body into a state of uncontrolled lust. Jerome is particularly picturesque in his revulsion against eating:

When that whole habitation of our interior man, stuffed with meats, inundated with wines, fermenting for the purpose of excremental secretion, is already being turned into a premeditatory of privies, where plainly nothing is so inevitable and natural as the savouring of lust.[20]

By the age of twenty-five, maybe a bit earlier, we are told, she (St Catherine of Siena) ate 'nothing' . . . While dressing the cancerous breast sores of a woman she was tending, Catherine felt repulsed at the horrid odor of the suppuration. Determined to overcome all bodily sensations, she carefully gathered the pus into a ladle and drank it all. That night she envisioned Jesus inviting her to drink the blood flowing from his pierced side, and it was with this consolation that her stomach 'no longer had need of food and no longer could digest' . . . Notwithstanding the vast differences between Catherine's drive to be united with God and the modern day anorexic's quest for a sense of self, the psychological dilemma is similar'.

From *Holy Anorexia* by Rudolph M. Bell

The women themselves were willing collaborators and colluded with the patriarchs to mortify their flesh. Today many of these women are acknowledged by the Catholic Church among their greatest saints. If they lived today, they would be recognised as anorexics and possibly be under enforced treatment. They fought food in the same way as the present-day anorexic woman and it held the same horrors. St Margaret Mary writes that she faced temptations against gluttony 'of which I had a greater horror than death'.[21] One of the greatest saints of all, and a Doctor of the Church, was Catherine of Siena, a terminal anorexic. She survived for long periods on Holy Communion alone, but she died before she was thirty, wasted and emaciated. She was seen by both lay people and clerics as a walking miracle and her life is still held up as an example of perfection to young Catholic girls. Nearly two thousand years after the beginning of this madness, women are still aspiring to 'perfection' in the same way.

DIETING AND RELIGION

I have received several letters from women who were, or have been, members of various evangelical churches. These letters told of the persecution they had suffered at the hands of their churches or ministers. They were told that they were sinners, that they *must* repent and lose weight. One woman even had the horrifying experience of being the subject of an exorcism:

> I was told that I was possessed by the demon of gluttony and of fat and that I must be delivered from it. The elders of the church held me down while others prayed over me to cast out the demon.

In Hillel Schwartz's marvellous book: *Never Satisfied: A Cultural History of Diets, Fantasies and Fat* Schwartz surveys the 20th-century religious diet mania in a chapter 'about extremes'. The first Christian diet book was called *Pray Your Weight Away* and was written by a Presbyterian minister who had lost 100 pounds and who said that 'we fatties are the only people on earth who can weigh our sin'. In 1967 another minister's offering was *Devotions for Dieters*, with helpful graces like

> I promise not to sit and stuff
> But stop when I have had enough. Amen.

Evelyn Kliewer invented 'The Jesus System For Weight Control' and in *Freedom from Fat* she proclaimed: 'With Jesus you can't lose — or should I say, all you *can* do is lose!' Another minister, C.S. Lovett, wrote *Help Lord — The Devil*

Wants Me Fat! and in the mid-1970s, Frances Hunter's *God's Answer to Fat – Lose it* sold more than 300,000 copies. Deborah Pierce had a 'Road to Damascus' conversion and prayed for deliverance from gluttony: 'The Lord is My Shepherd. He will lead me away from food and gluttony into higher paths of life.' Apparently, he did. By 1960 she was a top model in Washington and author of *I Prayed Myself Slim*.

As early as the 1950s there were religious slimming clubs in the United States. Deborah Pierce attended the Prayer-Diet Clubs to atone for her sin. Then there were the revivalist diet workshops led by a movement called Overeaters Victorious, who took as their motto a biblical text: 'He must increase but I must decrease' (John iii, 30), or (to quote yet another religious diet book title) *More of Jesus and Less of Me*. Carol Showalter, a minister's wife, saw a poster at a Weight Watchers meeting held in a Sunday-school room. It said 'Smile, God has the answer.' It appeared that Weight Watchers did not, for Mrs Showalter founded her own, Christian group, 3D — Diet, Discipline and Discipleship. [22]

I maintain that being fat is perceived as sin, both in the social and religious sense. Christians believe that Christ was crucified for their sins, and the *depth* and seriousness of the sin of fatness is made clear for us in Marie Capian's book about Overeaters Victorious: 'Jesus died on the cross for me to set me free from the addiction to wrong foods.' It is not difficult to make the link between these religious diet movements and slimming clubs or groups of a secular kind. The prevailing ethos is the same.

Church members in Nebraska went on a mass diet program 'offering their lard to the Lord'. Congregations competed for the most pounds lost in a 30 day period.

William J. Fabrey in *Radiance* Magazine, Winter 1990

Both Karen Armstrong[23] and Natalie Allon refer to the rituals of dieting as having strong religious undertones. The cult of dieting offers salvation and a new life. It can be as fanatical as born-again Christianity. The language is similar — fat equals sin, shame and failure, self-hatred and wickedness. Think of the terminology of slimming: 'I mustn't, I shouldn't, I've been wicked — naughty but nice, go on, be a devil, have just one. I've been really good this week. I feel a new person. I've left the old me behind.' In the course of my research for this book I found fat people described as transgressors, sinners, socially deviant, sick, irresponsible, weak-willed. The fat sinner sets out to become the thin saint.

Allon observes that group dieting accentuates the sinner-saint continuum. Meetings are structured on the lines of a fundamentalist church service. Individuals stand up and give testimonies as to their success or failure in the fight. Allon states that:

> Group dieting Believers discuss their faith in specific brands of diet creeds as technical aids to heal their fatness. Some offer testimonies to the Ideal of thinness as they talk about being born again or really living for the first time in their lives, now that they are on the road to salvation from their fatness sin. Prophetic group leaders offer sermons about the horrors of fatness and the evil fortunes which befall those who resist the dieting cure. The weekly offerings of recipe scripture passages show that there are enjoyable, even delicious ways to remain a saint-in-the-making and stick to the diet.[24]

Having been to Weight Watchers myself I can confirm this good-bad religiosity. It is powerful, containing elements of Catholicism as well as the fundamentalist approach. There is confession — the compulsory weigh-in each week and the giving account of any weight gained. A classic example is the Slimming World Clubs who measure food not in units or calories, but in Sin Values and some members call their manual 'The Bible'. There is penance in the form of having one's sins publicly pronounced and making a Firm Purpose of Amendment (determining to do better this week). And there is Absolution after real penitence has been shown.

In this way, the disapproval and punishment inflicted on the fat person by society are echoed and reinforced even within the 'support group'. Unless you lose weight you are seen as bad, a failure. One American writer calls diet groups a

> caricatured microcosm of the larger society chastising fatness as sin. The groups accentuate carefully nurtured self-hatred as a basis for salvation. The group dieter is made to feel that he or she is a psychological mess as a neurotically obese, depressive, anxious compulsive sinner. Group dieters condemn themselves for their need for immediate satisfaction, their inability to sustain frustration and the self-destructiveness of their over-eating. [25]

Persecution, then, of the fat person has a long and powerful history. The fact that it began with men who were afraid of women's sexuality is as relevant today as then. Women's flesh became synonymous with sexual temptation then, and now it is women who are the victims of prejudice and discrimination, far more than are fat men. In fact a fat man often carries good, wholesome images: look at Santa Claus, Mr Pickwick, Rumpole of the Bailey or Falstaff. A friend of mine is a fat — and extremely good — barrister. He told me:

> I could do with losing a few stones. But in my job, my size is an advantage. Presence is important and weight can

convey that. I can be an imposing figure in court whereas a weedy little barrister could be physically at a disadvantage. You need to be able to project yourself well to an audience of twelve across a distance of perhaps twenty yards. Barristers, on the whole, are not usually small, so if you are surrounded by other big blokes you are not going to feel out of place.

Men, in fact, need to make sure they maintain a *minimum* weight in order to be acceptable both to other men and to women. Everyone is familiar with the 'seven-stone weakling' jibe. Men are supposed to have rippling muscles, well-developed arms, legs and torsos: the admiring term 'he-man' has been replaced with 'macho'. Macho he-men are not thin, nor even slim. A thin woman is admired; a thin man brings the word 'weedy' springing to the minds if not the lips of those women who like their men to look like men (whatever that means). I have a couple of married friends. He is 6'2", she is 5'10". He is extremely thin and is the target of many a private snigger amongst the group they move in. She is also extremely thin, a size ten which at her height is very thin indeed. I have heard her called 'beautiful, elegant, enviably slim, able to wear anything'. She has no breasts but that does not matter. She is thin and she stays thin while she works out ways to cook meals that will help her skinny husband to put on weight.

I am not saying women can never be too thin, but it is unheard of for them to be mocked and jeered, much less penalised. Another friend is bone-thin. She is also greatly admired for her looks but admits she does sometimes feel self-conscious about her complete absence of female flesh. But it has never caused her problems, socially or sexually and she knows that when she walks into a crowded room the looks will be of admiration. The only thing that she feels is affected by her extreme thinness is her physical health.

SIZE AND THE WORKPLACE

Ten years ago Britain was not, on the whole, conscious of the blatant discrimination against people simply on account of their size. Persecution and prejudice yes, but denying people a job or promotion, or sacking them because they were fat? When such an incident was occasionally reported in the press it was a nine-day wonder. Yet it was happening all the time. In 1989, the magazine *What Diet and Lifestyle* ran a survey on discrimination. As many as 86 per cent of the respondents thought that fat people were discriminated against; 79 per cent believed that women were more discriminated against than men and 86 per cent felt that employers would favour a slim applicant for a job. In the United States, NAAFA collated the results of a huge survey and found overwhelming evidence of blatant discrimination at work. The respondents were divided into three categories: non-fat, moderately fat and fat. The incidence of discrimination was predictably high in the moderately fat group and very high in the fat group. Although the non-fat group did not report dismissal or denial of promotion, over 10 per cent were urged to lose weight at work and nearly 20 per cent were told to lose weight for unspecified medical reasons.

One of the conditions of your employment consists of maintaining a weight in harmony with your height.

Document for signature by Euro-Disney employees

Dismissing or refusing to hire a fat person is a piece of gross hypocrisy. British employers hide behind the Health and Safety Act or insurance requirements; yet many companies advertise that they are 'An Equal Opportunities Employer' and state in recruitment advertisements that they do not discriminate on the grounds of 'colour, gender, disability, sexual orientation or marital status'. Size, though is a different matter.

In 1988, Jane Meacham was working for Staffordshire County Council as a school dinner lady. She was dismissed on the medical officer's recommendation — he claimed that her obesity put her at risk from cardiac and muscular problems, and that overweight people were an economic liability as they took more time off through illness (this has never been proven or even indicated). Jane's story hit the tabloid headlines; 'Roly-Poly Dinner Lady Loses her Job' shouted *The Sun*. A journalist from that newspaper also telephoned Jane Meacham and asked if she would like their advice on weight loss! A television programme further highlighted the incident and the unfavourable publicity caused Staffordshire County Council to retract their decision and to announce that, in future, weight would not be taken into consideration. Jane declined to resume her post and got a job with a firm of industrial cleaners. Their medical adviser thought she should lose weight and she had to agree to do so in order to get the job. At 15 stones (210 lb) Jane Meacham was fit, healthy and athletic. She walked and swam regularly and followed a good balanced and nutritious diet.[26]

Britain has been apathetic in formulating any organised or legal defence against fat discrimination in spite of the increasing emphasis on employing those who have traditionally been oppressed. The Trades Union Congress will take action on behalf of its members and the Equal Opportunities Commission will take up cases of racial, sexual or gender discrimination. The only other law we have is that of unfair dismissal and that has to be negotiated by the individual. Needless to say, few fat people risk the heavy costs involved. A spokesman for the Institute of

Personnel Management pointed out that job applicants are at the mercy of the subjective judgement of the putative employer. The IPM says it does try to give guidelines to employers about choosing the right applicant for the job *regardless of appearance* but there is no way that these can be enforced.

In June 1989, a 34 year old divorced, disabled father of two was sentenced to lose 50 pounds in 90 days, or go to jail for failing to make child support payments. The judge called the decision 'his Oprah Winfrey sentence' and told reporters 'The only way this man will ever get back to being a productive worker is if he loses weight.'

NAAFA Newsletter, February 1990

I've been there myself. Working for the British Broadcasting Corporation, I found myself the target of two instances of size discrimination. I was told that my size precluded me from being considered as a newsreader for regional television, whatever my other qualities or qualifications for the job. And when working for Radio Four I was told by someone in high places, who said she 'meant well', that my talent was not being fully recognised or acknowledged because of my weight. On *radio*? 'It doesn't present a good image of the BBC when you go out on location,' said this woman. This, despite the fact that it was recognised that I had a good interviewing manner and personality and an ability to make interviewees feel at their ease. I rang the Equal Opportunities Commission who said they would act on the grounds of discrimination against appearance, but I'm sorry to say I did what I suspect most of us do. I kept quiet about it because I did not want to lose my job. I was never able to feel the same, though, and I left shortly afterwards.

While researching this book, I asked for women to write to me with their experiences of living as a fat woman in our society, including their experiences of discrimination. These are just a sample of incidences relating to employment or career:

I left university well-qualified and registered with an employment agency. Months went by, during which I just went from one job interview to the next. Finally one of the agency's recruitment counsellors told me that someone had put a note in my file to the effect that I was a pleasant person and with considerable ability but that because of my weight I would never get a job.

I'm a health visitor and I was told when applying for one job that they had so many applicants they didn't need to choose a fat one.

I was an assistant librarian and my boss was a fervent reformed dieter. She nagged and nagged at me to lose weight, even supervising my lunch hours, all the time with the threat that I would be made redundant if I didn't lose weight. I did lose a stone and a half very fast but it was a humiliating experience and I left.

I was working for Marks and Spencer and my contract came up for renewal. This meant I had to have a medical. Although I am fat I have always been healthy but my medical took place at the end of the day on Christmas Eve when it had been non-stop rush. My blood pressure was up — anyone's would have been. The doctor said that I was unlikely to get my contract renewed — word got round and I left before anything had been definitely decided — because there was so much pressure from my workmates to lose weight — I couldn't handle it.

I had an interview for a job as secretary in one of the top London hotels. I was told at the interview that I was not suitable, but the man interviewing me said that the hotel housekeeper had been on a very successful diet and would I like a word with her?

I went for a job as a secretary to a design company in East London and I had to *walk* right round the building so that the staff (male) could give me the 'once-over'. I was told very bluntly that the company had a certain image to maintain as they were in constant contact with the public, and it was suggested that I would not feel comfortable in this image. I wasn't offered the job, of course.

I saw an ad in an employment agency window for secretary to the editor of a fashion magazine. I was advised by the agency not to apply because of my size, and if I wanted to work for a magazine, then I would be better off applying to one of the slimming magazines. The agency even suggested I would have a good chance of getting a job as they could do a 'before and after' weight loss feature on me!

I am a singer and went for an audition at a local night-club. The vacancy was to 'fill the gap between two well-known artistes'. When I walked onto the stage I was told: 'Sorry — the gap isn't *that* big'.

During an economic recession the numbers of fat applicants being denied jobs increases. As one woman (already quoted) found — there are so many contending for each job that 'they don't need to choose a fat one'. The newspapers of the

1990s have been full of examples of size discrimination at work — but the issue no longer makes headlines or television news.

In June 1992, Britain's *Slimmer* Magazine published the findings of their survey into job discrimination. Some professions — such as airline cabin crew — automatically screen out overweight people, and not necessarily for the obvious reasons. According to *Slimmer*: '. . . the implication seems to be that as a rule, overweight people are sloppy individuals who don't care enough about their appearance — not British Airways material at all'. And nursing — traditionally a profession where you could expect to find large, comforting women — is now a no-entry area. They are told they will be unable to cope with the demanding physical work and that they will be at risk of back injury. *Slimmer* consulted Dr Stephen Pheasant, an ergonomist who has made a special study of body measurements (anthropometrics); he said that although research has shown that overweight people are *marginally* more likely to injure their backs, the extent of the increased likelihood is not known. I am sure a great number of those who have been hospitalised — especially if it was before about 1980 — will recall at least one fat nurse, who moved as quickly and did her job as efficiently as any of the thin ones. When I had my children (between 16 and 22 years ago) there was a senior midwife who was extremely fat, enormously respected, very efficient and hugely popular with patients and staff alike. This discrimination seems to me highly ironic in a profession known for its high rate of smokers, whose fitness is not questioned, I assume, as long as they are the right size.

In the United States the story is the same — though thanks to NAAFA (The National Association to Advance Fat Acceptance) size discrimination has been brought to the public consciousness for many years, and NAAFA has a long history of getting discriminatory policies reversed. This nationwide human/civil rights organisation was founded in 1969 by William Fabrey and Llewellyn Louderback. It was a much-needed reaction to fat oppression and size discrimination at all levels, and its purpose was — and is — 'to help fat people who', it contended, were 'the victims of prejudice, stigma, exclusion, exploitation and psychological oppression'. Bill Fabrey was not fat, but his own experience in applying for a job gave him what became an abiding interest in discrimination against fat people. As a skilled young electronics engineer, he applied to Eastman-Kodak, who had their own rules about weight. At the employment medical, Fabrey was told that he was 10 lb overweight at 12 stones and 5 pounds (175 lb). He was sent to the company dietitian but he refused to lose weight. Eastman-Kodak backed down, but only because there was an acute shortage of skilled people in this field. He contacted Llewellyn Louderback after reading a newspaper article by him entitled: 'More people should be Fat'.

Dulcie Plummer, a schools crossing attendant, or 'Lollipop Lady' in the north of England, was dismissed after a routine medical. She was told that she could only have her job back if she lost 2½ stones (35 lb). Mrs Plummer had done her job for 15 years during which time she had consistently weighed 15 stones (210 lb). When her employers, Nottingham Council, were asked for an explanation they admitted there was no reason for her dismissal and that she had always carried out her duties to everyone's complete satisfaction. An outcry from parents at the school concerned ensured that the incident reached the national press — and Mrs Plummer was reinstated immediately.

Being Fat Is Not A Sin

NAAFA is a powerful movement with chapters (regional groups) all over the United States. Its advisory board is an impressive line-up of physicians, attorneys and other relevant professionals, and it has assisted many fat people with discrimination law-suits. There are laws against size discrimination in Michigan State, Washington DC and Alameda County, California. In this last instance, change came about because of pressure put on the county authorities by just one woman, Louise Wolfe, an active member of NAAFA.

Airlines have particularly restrictive weight limits for flight attendants and there have been many mass lawsuits by cabin crew who have been sacked. One stewardess, Sherri Cappello was sacked for being 12 lb overweight — on the same day that she received her 25-year service badge. The company, American Airlines, was later forced to scrap the weight restrictions that cost Sherri Cappello her job, as a result of a case brought against them by the flight attendants' union and the Equal Employment Opportunity Commission. And in 1989, the now defunct PanAmerican World Airways agreed to pay $2.35 million to 116 female flight attendants who were disciplined, denied promotion, forced to resign or fired for being overweight.

With so many thousands of incidents of blatant discrimination, British and American fat women face humiliation at work all the time. NAAFA member Linda Karpenko was fired from her job at Hershey's, the confectionery manufacturers, towards the end of 1992 for 'insubordination'. Hershey's alleged that she did not follow safety regulations. Linda had been given a special chair to use during the course of her employment as the company claimed that sitting on an ordinary chair would pose a safety risk. Linda felt embarrassed and humiliated — she was not allowed to sit in any other chairs, but had to drag her own all over the building to attend meetings. This often entailed taking her chair along narrow corridors and into small elevators while her colleagues took their places in normal conference-room chairs. She refused to continue to drag her chair all over the building, so she was sacked. She has no money for a lawsuit but a trust fund has been set up for her and she intends to claim discrimination against Hershey Foods.[27]

The real feelings behind employment discrimination — those of revulsion and scorn — are conveniently hidden behind smokescreens like Health and Safety Acts. Donald Lennox, a former company chairman, spoke the truth: 'I don't like fat people. If I were recruiting and some guy waddled in with a big gut, he'd be dead before he opened his mouth.'

I could quote many sociological and psychological studies which prove that fat people are not considered worth employing; are perceived as lacking 'supervisory potential, self-discipline, professional appearance and personal hygiene'; where they are evaluated as 'significantly less competent, less productive, not industrious, disorganised, indecisive, inactive, less successful, less conscientious, less likely to take the initiative, less aggressive (I would call that a plus!), less likely to persevere at work, less ambitious, more mentally lazy and less self-disciplined than average-weight or underweight subjects. But Donald Lennox puts it much more succinctly. That is what we are up against. People who want us dead. Don't think that the eugenic dream died with Hitler. It is alive and well in the minds of fat-haters.

SIZE AND THE MEDICS

Llewellyn Louderback remarked that advising a fat person to see his physician is like telling a mouse to go see a cat. With some rare exceptions, I agree with that. Dr Esther Rothblum, an associate professor of psychology at the University of Vermont in the United States, is a fat woman who has concentrated her research in the area of stigmatisation against the overweight. Speaking at the 1992 NAAFA Convention, she quoted extensive studies she had carried out on the various types of prejudice which showed that doctors and other health-care professionals were among the worst offenders. 'We received the most horrendous examples of (medical) discrimination,' she said. 'People did not just say: "My doctor told me to lose weight", people said things like: "My doctor said if he had a dollar for every pound I was overweight he could pay off his mortgage"; "My doctor said I might as well buy a gun and shoot myself"; "My doctor said I couldn't get pregnant, I was fat, who would want to make me pregnant (and it turned out I was pregnant)". In her speech, Esther Rothblum called these incidents: 'Tremendous examples of malpractice, not just harassment or kindly meant advice'.

Studies of doctors' attitudes to their overweight patients have consistently demonstrated that they are an extremely prejudiced group. One study shows that doctors dislike fat people, and that this dislike comes from their own middle-class values rather than from their training or from any scientific basis. The doctors in the study preferred not to manage the overweight patient and most did not. They did not expect success when they treated the overweight, and believed it to be unaesthetic and indicative of a lack of personal control. The doctors surveyed gave an extremely negative picture of the very overweight person, describing them as weak-willed, ugly and awkward. They evaluated them more harshly than the overweight patients evaluated themselves and this gives a clear indication of the extent of their prejudice as fat people are known to have extremely low self-esteem, acting as a mirror of society's judgement. The fat patient is at the mercy of the doctor who very often sees no reason to treat this deviant with the respect and basic good manners that he would normally accord someone.

Social mores seem to go out of the window and the fat person is soon aware that she is a wrong-doer — once again, a sinner.[28]

When I was researching this book I was intrigued by what doctors would confide to me on the telephone, not knowing that I, too, was one of their deviants. In this way, I learnt that physicians really do resent having to waste skill and time on a patient whom they considered walking proof that she would not take steps to restore herself to a state of normalcy when it was (apparently) within her power. The general consensus was that any physical condition was harder to treat because of the prevailing overweight, and even helping their patients to lose weight was unrewarding because of the very high incidence of recidivism. I am not castigating the entire medical profession in one fell swoop; there are of course, exceptions, including my own doctor.

Not so a former doctor. When I visited him because I was anxious that my one-year-old child would not eat solid food in any form, I received the sneering response: 'What are you trying to do? Make the child as fat as yourself?' Or the midwife who came into the labour ward minutes after I had given birth, suspended in a haze of elation and exhaustion, sharply aware of the narrow divide between life and death which is so often brought home to women during childbirth: 'You do realise you're going to die an early death?' I was told while she was checking the placenta.

Like many women, I have experienced the eager desire to please the doctor by losing weight. It is not a personal desire to please; rather, an attempt to gain a degree of respect and caring normally denied us but there if we prove that we can show self-control. It is very difficult to stand up to doctors because there is the fear underneath that if we displease them too much they could refuse us some vital, life-saving help. That if we were to call them out with frightening chest pains, they might sit and finish their crossword first because we might not be worth helping.

Paranoid fantasy? On the whole I hope it is, but it is born of the bewilderment that comes from a lifetime of being spoken to rudely, hurtfully, without respect or consideration or acknowledgement of the full extent of the fat person's humanity. And it can strike unexpectedly. Recently I had to have a D&C. I'd put it off because I dreaded that vulnerable feeling of being in hospital unable to protect myself or retaliate against the insults. I was lucky in having a woman consultant, who saw me in clinic and arranged to do the operation herself under local anaesthetic. In hospital she brought me a form to sign on the morning of the operation. I read it; it stated that I gave consent to any operative procedures that were considered necessary including the administration of a general anaesthetic. I crossed out that bit, because I am allergic to general anaesthetic (nothing to do with my weight) and signed the form. My consultant turned from being an understanding friend into a fury. I was not allowed to cross things out, she said officiously and made it clear that her anger was because she construed my altering of the form as a lack of trust in her — it was nothing to do with the fact that I was fat as that had not been an issue that had concerned her. Or so it had seemed. Even she could not resist a jibe. 'They wouldn't give *you* a general anaesthetic anyway,' she said with contempt.

In the survey I conducted of over two hundred fat women and their feelings and experiences, the question about doctors hit many raw nerves. Again and again women reported fear of going to the doctor because of the lectures about their weight:

Every time I go, he nags me about my weight — it doesn't matter what I'm there for. I could break my arm and he'd say it was because I'm too fat.

Three years ago I started having pains in my chest and shortness of breath. The doctor immediately said that I must lose weight and I was so frightened that I did. In the next couple of weeks I had all the tests for heart disease and they found nothing wrong. I kept having bouts of pain and in the end they diagnosed it as stress-related, even muscular. But I was made to feel that if anything was wrong with my heart it was all my fault, self-inflicted and therefore not worth being helped.

I found a lump in my breast and my doctor asked me to wait in his surgery while he wrote a letter to a specialist. I saw him write 'This grossly obese patient reports . . .' and I said to him 'Why are you putting that? It isn't relevant and anyway the specialist will be able to see my size for himself'. He had the grace to admit the description wasn't necessary and he started the letter again. But it upset me to think that I wasn't just a patient in his mind, I was a 'grossly obese' patient.

I've got a gastric ulcer which my doctor blames on my weight. I cannot find any evidence that overweight causes ulcers, but I feel that there is an element of bargaining in the treatment she gives me — if I will be 'good' and lose weight she will be more sympathetic, but until I do . . .

I'd been having heavy periods (I eventually had a D&C which fixed them) and my doctor said they would improve if I lost weight. He even put me on Ponderax which I know most GP's don't use now because it is an amphetamine. I lost the weight but it didn't stop the trouble. I stopped taking the Ponderax because I felt terrible and the weight just came back.

I don't go to the doctor. I avoid it whenever possible. Only if it's life or death. I'm too scared to go to the doctor.

Lin, who had the episodes of chest pain, and Sian with the lump in her breast both talked about the 'nightmare' effects of having something wrong with them that was possibly life-threatening, combined with the feeling that somehow they could not expect the support reserved for 'normal' patients. The elements of being a sinner were strongly felt — and also something close to a feeling that they were being treated as though they had cried 'wolf' — something to do with the apparent lack of real importance attached to their symptoms.

But by far the most shocking and terrifying example of the effect of the medical profession's hatred of us was a bleak and hopeless cry from an American woman:

> Being fat is going to kill me, not because of the strain on my heart but because of the strain on my soul. I am going to have some warning signs and avoid seeking health care until it is too late, because I am sick and tired of the canned speeches from doctors and nurses blaming my weight for everything.

This was said in a therapy group led by Angela Barron McBride, Associate Dean of the Indiana School of Nursing, and was quoted by Karl Niedershuh in the *Philadelphia Daily News*.[29] Niedershuh's 34-year-old wife, Cindy, died in June 1990 after an operation which she came through without problems. A few days later she suffered a pulmonary embolism — a blood clot that lodges in the lungs, and she died. Cindy had had a pituitary tumour for 18 years. The pituitary is the 'master' gland in the body and if it is affected, the endocrine system goes haywire. Among other things, growth is affected and Cindy was unable to prevent her body from getting fatter, until at the end of her life she weighed more than 500 lb.

Karl Niedershuh describes how her tumour remained untreated because the diagnostic equipment was not big enough to support Cindy. She got shunted from doctor to doctor, none of whom was able to treat the disease but most of whom were keen to put her on a diet. One specialist endocrinologist dismissed her when she refused to take the Medifast low-calorie diet programme at the hospital. A few — mostly young — doctors did show sympathy and respect, and one found her a scanner capable of taking her size. It was only when she finally had the scan, which produced an image — proof of her condition — that she was accepted for surgery.

Karl was more than aware of the risks. But in the hospital cafeteria he heard orderlies making jokes and comments about his wife. When Cindy died, doctors told him that emboli are more common in large patients. This is true — but it is also true that blood clots, or thrombosis, is a recognised hazard of any operation, *whatever size* the patient. The condition is prevented by early mobility as soon as possible after surgery, and by the use of special bandages on the legs to prevent the formation of a thrombosis. Even when a patient cannot immediately get up, physiotherapists give leg-moving exercises which can be done lying in bed. Karl Niedershuh questions why his wife was not treated with the kind of 'aggressive action' which could have prevented the clot, especially as her size made her more susceptible. He feels she was 'killed by sheer indifference. It was easier to just ignore her, and put "obesity" on her death certificate.'

I was moved to tears by Karl Niedershuh's article. Tears of anguish for him and Cindy, and of anger at the doctors and health-care workers who caused her such physical, mental and emotional suffering, and who laughed and jeered and made obscene jokes about her size. There is no self-pity in Karl's account. Just the most immense suffering, and love. He says of his 500-lb wife: 'She was, without question, the most beautiful woman I have ever known. She brought more love and caring into the world in her 34 years that most of us could imagine in seventy.'

Having said all this — and it needed saying — I am glad to be able to report that there are exceptions. Dr Fran Watson of Minneapolis noticed that her fat patients tended to be healthy, and this led her to question the perceived medical wisdom on the links between obesity and poor health. She started advising her patients that they need not lose weight as long as they were active, healthy and eating well. Fran Watson expresses great concern about the effect of doctors' negative and condemning attitudes towards fat patients because the fear of seeing a doctor can lead to problems going undiagnosed. As a medical underwriter for the National American Life and Casualty insurance company, she is also aware of the difficulty a fat person faces in finding health insurance. She advises going to a broker who will find a company with a more enlightened and liberal attitude to weight than is usual. Her own company insures supposedly high-risk clients; people who have had open-heart or bypass surgery, and certainly 'the larger person'.

Both Britain and the United States have the cult of 'media doctors', who in many ways are even more influential than our own GPs because of their celebrity status. Britain's Dr Miriam Stoppard, always a diet advocate, has a persuasive personality and an air of sincerity which gives the viewing public great faith in her diet books. The United States has its share of similar personalities — but it also has Dr Dean Edell, a medical journalist internationally syndicated in print and on television, who frequently speaks and writes about size discrimination and the myths about fat people. In a four-part television series on dieting. Dr Edell gave viewers some essential facts to counteract widely prevalent myths, most of which are perpetuated by doctors themselves:

There is a genetic predisposition to weight retention that has been proven in studies of twins.

It is possible to be both fat and fit through the proper selection of food groups and with the right amount of exercise.

Fat people, as a group, eat no more than thin people, as a group.

Fat people, as a group, have no more illness than thin people, as a group.

He also pleads with yo-yo dieters to 'stop undermining their health and self-esteem with a practice that only makes them fatter'. He recommends that fat people keep up to date with medical research, and suggests they challenge their doctors with the facts; for instance 'Doctor, don't you read the New England Journal of Medicine?' (or whatever is applicable), 'Haven't you seen the studies that say there are a lot of people like me who don't eat excessively, who are fat and can be healthy? I find your comments discriminatory. And obnoxious.' Edell says: 'People have to educate the medical profession. It's going to be a long, uphill battle.'

Where doctors are concerned, it is worth rehearsing a few words to say next time you are told that you must lose weight; perhaps just saying that you are aware of your weight, that you have not visited the doctor or hospital because of it and that you do not require advice about it, would suffice. And you might suggest that if the doctor has a problem caring for fat patients, maybe he could recommend someone else who would not feel quite so strongly.

In 1990 I moved house and out of the catchment area of my doctor with whom I had felt safe for years. She was non-judgemental, did not attribute any illness to my weight, and was more concerned about the deleterious effects of dieting. It was quite frightening having to find a new doctor, but I had written this book and knew I could practise what I had preached, as it were. I registered with several doctors before I found one I was happy with. I asked each doctor for his or her opinion on whether or not I should be encouraged to diet; or whether my weight would be responsible for any condition I might develop; if his or her judgement and/or treatment might be prejudiced or in any way different from that offered to a patient of average weight. They were either honest in their responses, or I detected from the way in which they replied whether they had a personal ethos which would be influenced by my weight. I found a woman doctor in the next town with all the qualities a fat woman needs and who makes it her business to keep up to date with research. It *can* be done; you *have* to remember that doctors are flawed, fallible human beings.

We may not have a Dr Dean Edell in Britain, but when this book was first published, I did see signs of hope. I expected a torrent of 'hate mail' from outraged doctors; I received a number of letters from doctors saying that they supported what I had written, or that it had made them realise that they had treated their 'overweight' patients badly. This is an example:

I am currently working in general practice and I blush at the memory of occasions when I must have inflicted horrible psychological wounds on my maligned overweight patients. Nevertheless I am trying to make recompense and I have become involved in a study that the stigma attached to overweight has a negative effect on my patients' well being.

PREGNANCY

Pregnancy is the area where women seem to feel most vulnerable. Anyone who has been pregnant will know the feeling of trusting their baby's safety to the experts and will do anything to ensure this. In addition the pregnant woman is particularly sensitive to hostility or negativity because that in itself appears to contain some kind of threat to her or her baby's well-being. Antenatal visits occur once a month, becoming more frequent as the pregnancy progresses. Each visit entails being weighed and having the baby palpated through the abdomen. Very often this procedure is performed by students. Until they are familiar with what the different parts of the baby feel like through the abdominal wall, palpation is not easy for students and it is obviously more difficult if there is more than a thin layer of fat between their examining hands and the fluid-encased foetus. So a fat woman, lying helpless and undignified on her back, is the butt of jokes and jeers by all but the relatively small number of sensitive and thoughtful doctors. Dawn was to have her baby in a teaching hospital: 'One day the doctor was examining me with a lot of students watching. That was embarrassing enough, but the doctor said "Look at all this — what do you think you're going to give birth to, an elephant?"'

When Dawn became pregnant she weighed sixteen stones; after her daughter was born she put off having another baby, feeling unable to face the humiliation that had been a constant part of her first pregnancy. Eventually she decided that she could not go through with it again, and her daughter remains an only child. Several women I spoke to felt that the treatment they received by doctors and midwives in pregnancy and labour was the reason they only had one child. [30]

With my first pregnancy, I came to dread the antenatal visits and the snide remarks every time I was weighed or examined. There was only one way I could cope with them, and I proceeded to lose weight. Each visit after that found my weight was stable: what the pregnancy put on in weight I lost from my body. It earned approval and respect from the hospital staff and I felt I then 'deserved' to ask questions about my pregnancy and to make specific requests for the sort of labour I wanted. I was not very overweight when I was expecting my second baby and it felt quite different — I was congratulated for having lost so much since the first one and I basked in the pleasure of being treated normally. By the time my third pregnancy had begun I had put all the weight back on, plus some more and it was a nightmare — from the very first examination by the family planning doctor to confirm pregnancy ('I sincerely hope you're not pregnant at that weight,' she said before examining me, and on finding that indeed I was, she walked out of the room in disgust, leaving me to dress and remove myself) to the discovery that I had a hormone deficiency which required twice weekly injections from the district nurse. Being pregnant and at the mercy of one's hormones induces mood swings in the best of circumstances. My memory of that pregnancy is of the district nurse haranguing me each time she came to my house to give me the injections, while I stood with tears pouring down my face, almost begging her to stop going on about the risks of being pregnant at my weight; after all I *was* pregnant. You become a supplicant in these situations — there was only one answer that I could see and once again I started to lose weight during my pregnancy.

I am quite aware that much of this may sound like a litany of complaint, self-pity on my part and on the part of those women who confided to me their painful experiences. We are wide open to criticisms of 'whingeing'. The fact is, and it *is* a fact, that a great deal of real pain and fear is experienced by women when they put themselves, with their fat bodies, in the hands of doctors and obstetricians. There can be no doubt that we are seen as sinners and criminals and, unless we display signs of penitence and penance by losing weight, we stand convicted.

We need to have the courage of Margaret who presented herself at the hospital, newly pregnant, very overweight, over forty and with eight children already. First a termination was suggested, then when she refused it was suggested that at her age and vast weight the pregnancy was dangerous. Margaret, lying on an examination couch, stripped of her identity with the shedding of her clothes and wearing a too-small hospital gown wasn't having any of this:

> I sat bolt upright and just glared at them, I was so angry. Then I said: 'It is your job to see that my baby is born safely and that I receive the best possible care in pregnancy. That is why I am here'. It worked.

In the past I have walked into a doctor's surgery or a hospital consulting room with a smile and placatory words such as: 'Look, I know I'm overweight but I *am* doing something about it — I am following a diet and am losing X pounds a week (or have lost X pounds or stones).' I have said this whether it is true or not, and I am an articulate person. What happens to the woman who is abused for her weight and does not have the courage, the education, the background to enable her to fight back? There is still this air of 'mystique' surrounding the medical profession, and the 'doctor knows best' attitude prevails even with the educated middle classes. For the working-class woman it is much harder to refute what the doctor says so she is more inclined to take her pain within herself and absorb the insults without comment.

The power to heal, to save lives is invested with magical qualities and lay people are responsible for allowing doctors to maintain the God Almighty complexes that so many of them have. It is not entirely their fault if we pander to their vanity and to their apparent omniscience and omnipotence.

TOO FAT TO BE A MOTHER

Discrimination does not stop in the workplace, though. It can invade and shatter the private lives of people who are singled out for their imperfections, their crime against what can only be called the fascism in society. In 1984, the British press reported the case of Mrs Inger Johannson of Vaggeryd in Sweden, who was given an ultimatum by social welfare officers — to lose weight or lose her child. Rune Berg, chief of the local social services, claimed 'concern' that Mrs Johannson's weight would cause problems for her three-year-old son when he started school. The boy would be picked on, he said, because his mother was obese. Inger Johannson was reported as 'Living in perpetual fear of someone coming to the door to take her son away'. Mrs Johannson, who weighed 17st. 13 lb was told to go to a health farm to lose weight, or have her child taken into care.

On the other side of the world, an Australian couple, Michael and Susie Murnane, tried to adopt an abandoned baby from Sri Lanka. They met all the requirements of the Sri Lankan government services except one. They were considered too fat. Susie Murnane, at 14st. 7 lb, was ordered to reduce to 10st. 3 lb, and her husband, who was 14st. 2 lb, was told to lose a proportional amount. The Sri Lankan government, along with several other Third World countries like South Korea, imposes a maximum weight on every adoptive parent. The justification for this is that fat people supposedly have a greater risk of ill-health and the child would therefore be more likely to lose a parent.

In a country like Sir Lanka the babies like the one the Murnanes applied to adopt are part of a vast army of homeless, parentless waifs. It seems nonsense to turn down prospective parents on the grounds of overweight, especially as the health risks are not proven. Fortunately in this case, the absurdity was realised and the couple were allowed to adopt after all.

The American Sate of Wisconsin deemed Barbara and Gordon Ray unsuitable to adopt a baby because they were too fat. They had a good deal to offer a baby — they owned their house, they were employed, their doctor pronounced them in good health and they both had a family history of obesity *and* longevity, and it is medically recognised that family history is a truer indicator than weight itself. Mrs Ray is 5'9" and weighs fifteen stones and Mr Ray at 6'2" weighs nearly sixteen. With their heights that is not vastly overweight by any definition — except that of the insurance companies, the advertising industry, the dieting industry and all those other profit-making concerns.[31] The Rays were lucky to be living in Wisconsin, because the state governor overruled the decision not to let them adopt. He said his grandmother had been fat, and had suffered no ill effects on account of it.

But perfectly suitable young American couples are being turned down because of their size, even if they can prove good health. NAAFA members recommend networking — keeping eyes and ears open for a chance to adopt privately. It is illegal to advertise to adopt a child. Some adoption agencies have been found to be less restrictive than most (addresses from NAAFA at the back of this book). NAAFA itself has drawn up a policy on adoption, targeting the media, adoption agencies, child-welfare workers, and others who mistakenly believe that size makes a person unfit to be a parent. NAAFA also offers support to those facing discrimination in this matter, and will assist with litigation by providing referrals to expert witnesses who could testify on behalf of the couples or individuals attempting to adopt a child.

This is a particularly cruel form of discrimination as well as being utterly ridiculous. It is a form of totalitarianism that makes you wonder what will come next — compulsory abortion for fat pregnant women, perhaps.

What about Britain, where there is an acute shortage of babies for adoption? The British Agencies for Adoption and Fostering do give their prospective adopting parents a thorough medical. They made the point that fat people could be 'marvellous with teenagers' but they might not be chosen for young children or babies.[32] The Agencies' social worker looks into the life-styles of obese would-be adopters in the same way as they do with the disabled. She might turn up at a meal time to check dietary habits, to ensure that the family was not sitting round eating chip butties or boxes of chocolates, and to try to see if the 'problem' was emotionally linked.

What actually happens is that the overweight ones tend to become the foster parents as this does not require a medical. Although not stated, the chances of a substantially fat woman being allowed to adopt a baby are slight,[33] and this is borne out by countless fat people who are turned down as adopting parents.

Barnardos also admitted to overweight foster parents but showed hesitation over a fat woman adopting a baby. The reasons given were couched in concern about mobility, the difficulties of lifting children, or the ability to keep up with a hyperactive child,[34] which is patently nonsense and is based on the myths that fat people cannot be fit, together with the prejudice which labels us as slow, ineffectual and lumbering.

Discrimination which states overtly or otherwise, 'You are not wanted because you are undesirable, ugly, lazy, inefficient' is vindictive. But the less direct kind of prejudice, masquerading as concern for the welfare of others, in this case children, is even more insidiously threatening. The only way to fight it is to bring it out into the open and question it. We should arm ourselves with facts about fat women's health and quote them at those who profess concern for our well-being when they urge us to lose weight or bar doors to us. We should be asking questions about the treatment given to other 'health risk' groups: do those who deem us unfit to work, to appear on television, to adopt children apply the same criteria to smokers? Or to the very underweight?

3
Dying to be thin and developing a fat personality

No man shall know me
I shall not touch bread
I will dance, I will dance
Till I'm dead.

Two raw cauliflowers, two black puddings,
one and a half pounds of raw liver, two pounds of kidneys,
a piece of cheese,
three pounds of raw carrots, two pounds of peas,
a pound of mushrooms, ten peaches, four bananas,
two apples,
four pears,
two pounds of plums,
two pounds of grapes
and some home-made bread.

She lay beached
Her belly
swelling
Cradled in arms
already whittled
To a skeleton.
No child grew
Under hollow breast
She died by her own hand
And mouth.

This poem was written by a British teacher, Clare Dannatt, in memory of Pauline Seaward, a model and dancer who died in 1981 after an eating binge.

The food listed in the poem was eaten in one go; almost impossible to imagine in terms of sheer quantity. The mind revolts at the idea of the stomach being able to accommodate the volume. But more bizarre and incomprehensible than the food itself is the state of mind Pauline must have reached to commit such a suicidal act — and one in which she did not die a quick or painless death.

In the mid 1920s, the author of a diet book confidently predicted that the law would eventually 'make excess avoirdupois a misdemeanor, if not a high crime, punishable by compulsory shoe-shining, tight corsets, or some other suitable form of discomfort.

From *Fat Power* by Llewellyn Louderback

Hers is an extreme example, a horrifying, shocking and almost unbelievable response to the demands of a warped culture. Pauline was a dancer and a model so her life was one of constant vigilance, monitoring every calorie, every inch and every ounce of weight gained or lost. She was highly visible in her profession and control was the essence of her life-style.

It is not relevant to discuss whether Pauline Seaward was anorexic, bulimic, or to use the American term, bulimarexic, a combination of both. What her death illustrates profoundly and tragically is the consequence of years of tautly maintained control over her natural eating patterns and perhaps her natural weight.

Novelist Marge Piercy tells of a dinner party where the hostess made one of the guests stand up and announced to the gathering that 'Nancy has lost 20 lb. Isn't that fabulous!' Marge Piercy says she was shocked as Nancy stood and everyone applauded. The woman in question had recently had an exhibition of paintings at a prestigious gallery. A doctor present had built a house with his own hands and Piercy herself had finished a novel that had taken seven years of research. These accomplishments, she says, were not deemed worthy of applause, but for Nancy 'having caused part of her body to disappear seemed to everyone else in the room an act of such singular merit it overwhelmed the merely artistic or commercial success.'[1]

Doctors are reporting a frightening new drug trend — girls and young women using highly addictive cocaine and crack to lose weight. According to an article in the *Los Angeles Times*, there is a new 'misguided but growing perception that it is a quick, cheap and easy way to lose weight. Drug dealers are even promoting these dangerous drugs with this in mind. A ten-year-old girl from New York reported being approached by a dealer who told her that boys only like thin girls.'

Quoted in NAAFA Newsletter, December 1990

I once belonged to a small, smart and very professional Early Music Group. For the recitals we gave, usually in rather splendid places like ornate chapels and Bishops' palaces, we were required to wear a 'uniform' of long black velvet skirt and pintucked white blouse. Because the music we sang was very beautiful it was required that we should try and match it. I continually fought a battle with myself to stay in the group — I loved the singing but hated the feeling of being an outcast, especially at concerts. There were only five other women so it was impossible not to stand out. Then one year I had been on one of my diets and lost a considerable amount of weight. With great pride I made a huge tuck in the waistband of my skirt and fastened it with a nappy pin — I'm no needlewoman. And I bought a new white blouse from Marks and Spencer which had previously been off limits — I had only been able to buy clothes in Evans Outsize as they were then called.

There was no doubt — I felt so much more confident as I stood with the group in front of an audience. I felt I belonged fully in a way that I had not before. And the picture in the local paper showed me blending with the group, not standing out as usual. It is hard to deny the relief and pleasure I felt during that period of comparative slimness. When you lose weight people tend to treat you as though you have returned to the human race, and there is never any shortage of encouragement. 'You've lost weight!' people cry. And then comes the conspiratorial bit: 'Don't you *feel* much better? You know, you look *years* younger. You should feel very proud of yourself — you deserve to.' The message is loud and clear, she that was lost has been found and returned to the fold — the parable of the lost sheep and the prodigal son all in one, except that the weight-loser will be more likely to be welcomed back with a plate of nouvelle cuisine than a fatted calf.[2]

As you challenge the assumption that thin is the only way to be beautiful, you not only change your own belief, you can slowly reshape long-standing cultural attitudes too. In doing so you'll help make this society a happier and healthier place for people of every size and shape.

Rita Freedman, psychologist, quoted in *Radiance*, Fall 1990

With that kind of yardstick, and it is not rare, it is completely unsurprising that fat women find social situations painful, for the same voices that congratulate the dieter are those that imply or overtly state condemnation of the fat sinner. The following is a sample from the letters I have received:

I don't eat or drink at parties because of the remarks: 'Don't eat that, it'll make you fat'.

I don't go to swimming baths because of the comments: 'Make way for Moby Dick' was one of them.

Your size will be over there (Grannies' department).

I was in a restaurant and the waitress said 'Try our special grilled fish with a lovely crisp salad'.

Oh God — changing in communal fitting rooms.

Getting in and out of low cars when people are watching.

I'm embarrassed at going on things in fairgrounds, like those swinging chairs — I'm scared the chains will break.

I drink *before* I go to a party to settle my nerves about feeling out of it.

I went on holiday to Spain and hated every minute of it — I didn't feel I could wear a swimming costume or strapless tops.

A complete stranger, a weedy Sloane, once stopped in the street at the sight of me in one of my African print caftans and brayed, wonderingly, 'Don't you think you're a little OVERWEIGHT?'.

I went to a health farm to try and lose some weight and in spite of the fact that that's what they're supposed to be all about I was too embarrassed to mix with the other guests who were all slim or slightly overweight. I felt grotesque wearing a tracksuit and swimming costume and I couldn't enjoy the massages because I felt they must be hating my body.

I love disco dancing and although I am very fat I think I have good movement and rhythm. I was determined not to give up something I enjoyed and I used to go and dance, ignoring all the stares and sniggers. But I stopped because I found it too stressful being laughed at.

My daughter's wedding. All the the guests were so slim and beautifully dressed. Worst of all was the family group photos — *his* mother is an elegant, tall size 12.

We came to live here when I was fifteen — I'm from Jamaica. I was very plump, not huge, but I had no idea that it was unacceptable in Britain. No one had ever mentioned losing weight back home, it was unheard of. So for a time I stayed myself, but I couldn't cope with being black *and* fat. I've dieted because I want to be acceptable at school, parties, discos and I want a boyfriend. But it's very hard to lose the weight and keep it off.

Random samples of women's everyday feelings and experiences; many of the same kind were reported by a large number of women. The critic will scoff at the apparent triviality of such incidences. To play devil's advocate, I could say that these women are whingeing, attaching importance to minor grouses. Think of all the people much worse off — think of those in wheelchairs, and after all, if we don't like being ostracised, we can do something about it, can't we? The pain of being socially disadvantaged and outcast is great. It permeates a person's entire being. As one woman sums up her observation at being fat out in society:

> We all recognise the 'looks' from other people, and know so well what they mean. The double-take, the hurried averting of eyes, the frankly boggle-eyed stare, the nudge to draw a companion's attention, the ill-stifled sniggers, the muttered astonishment of disgust, the hurried shushing of the loud and frank remarks of a young child, the disdainful sneer of the very slim (who may have only just achieved that status), the pitying 'Oh, the poor thing' look on the face of the kindly mumsy lady; all these are to me, more hurtful in their way than open rejection or discrimination.

Fat women are not masochists — they hurt. If they could 'do something about it' wouldn't they? Wouldn't we? Those — and I indict the majority of the medical profession — who attach blame to the overweight individual and penalise them accordingly, need to stop for a moment and ask themselves *why* that woman puffing as she runs for a bus doesn't help herself by shedding a couple of stones. The doctor who shakes his head when a woman presents herself with severe backache should ponder before he pontificates about what can she expect carrying round all that excess weight. Why do we do this to ourselves? It is so much *easier* to be slim. An American once said that a woman striving for recognition in the achievement-oriented world of careers at the top has to be twice as good as a man in order to be thought half as good. This is doubly true of fat women, not just in the professional but in the social world. To be taken seriously the fat woman needs to make twice the effort of the slim one.

The public is ill-informed about weight, dieting and weight loss. Shamefully, physicians are often no better informed. In researching this book I spoke to about a dozen experts in the field of obesity treatment and asked them a simple question: *How* can fat women become slim? When they had considered all the diets and surgery the answer was that the majority cannot. And it is a huge majority too, 98 per cent. Yes, people can lose weight — and in enormous amounts — but it is invariably regained and the research currently going on has not yet come up with the answer to the simple question, fired thousands of times a day at thousands of women: Why don't you lose weight?

When fat women appear on television, defending their right to be as they are and to be left alone, they are often asked a question by the interviewer: 'If you could take a pill that would make you slim overnight would you do so?' These women are realists and they know they have to live in a tough hostile world. They may have come to terms with their size because they have learnt and accepted that dieting does not work. But they are not martyrs or masochists. Why should they opt for the hostility? So their answer is invariably 'Yes.' As mine would be. Except that I would qualify my answer — I would not like to be slim as I do not think it would suit me and I like being an Earth Mother. I would like a magic pill to make me less fat and to ensure that I stayed that way.

But if I am talking about being socially acceptable then surely any degree of fat would exclude me? Yes and no is the only and complex answer to that. Women's response to outside pressure to conform is variable. I believe there are as many reasons for being fat as there are fat women. Each woman's body, eating patterns and size are her own, laid down before birth, or formed by the physical and psychological experiences of her life. And it is those experiences which determine the way a woman feels about her body. At the very end of the scale there is the anorexic whose body-image is so distorted she perceives normal weight as grotesquely fat and lives in fear of 'normality'. One of the unhappiest letters I received was from Anne, a woman weighing eleven and a half stones at 5'2" and a size 18. It is clear from Anne's letter that every aspect of her life is blighted by her unhappiness about her weight. She 'feels a complete failure.' She cannot bring herself to go to parties, or swimming or disco dancing, two of her favourite activities. She went through a stage of being promiscuous, which she now deeply regrets, but did so out of a need to feel needed. She has written to Claire Rayner for help but cannot take her advice to 'accept herself as she is'. To a size 12 happily within the social limits, Anne's size and weight might be perceived as grotesque. To me, knowing I look and feel good at twelve stones, I'd swap places with her tomorrow! So why this tremendous range of relativity?

I think it has many roots. Anne went on local radio and did a sponsored slim with other women — she was the winner, achieving the best and quickest weight loss. She put all the weight back on a month after the programme finished. The clue to her present unhappiness lies in her feelings about that period:

> I felt fantastic at 10st. 4 lb (144 lb). God, it was such a struggle, I ate seven hundred calories per day and did the most strenuous exercises imaginable. I also walked two miles every day. When I put it on again I felt such a failure and I still do.

The key word is failure. Fat women have failed — to conform to the rules of the society and culture we live in; to meet and measure up to social, medical and media standards set for us; to live up to our own expectations of ourselves; to harness qualities like self-control, pride, will-power — the litany is almost limitless.

Anne's success at attaining a weight that felt good is perceived as ridiculous by Helen who is nine stones (126 lb) at 5'2". Helen wants to weigh seven and a half stones (105 lb) (the acceptable average for her height as given in the Metropolitan Life Insurance tables is eight stones (112 lb)) but Helen is small-boned and feels she should weigh less than average for her height. At nine stones (126 lb) she looks slim and has no weight problems. Yet she considers herself a stone and a half (21 lb) overweight and 'could not bear the thought of being any heavier'.

Maureen is a size 18 at 5'5" and does not find clothes a problem. She would not worry very much about her weight were it not for the fact that Weight Watchers have pronounced her 'about five stones overweight'. This is patently ridiculous, but such is the power of the word of God as personified by the slimming clubs that Maureen has been brainwashed into believing she is massively overweight. Again, there are many large women who would envy Maureen's 'weight problem' but the fact is that her perception of herself has been shaped by the chastening effect of being pronounced imperfect — and by a wide margin — so she too feels a failure:

My confidence in my physical appearance is almost nil. Mirror avoidance is a hobby of mine — I loathe my shape and my own ability to do something about it. I'd love to be slim but it will only happen if my will-power strengthens sufficiently to see me through five stones of dieting.

Who says what is fat? And who decrees what degree of fat is too fat? Those questions are not as rhetorical as they may sound. It would appear that there is a fine line between being fat and unacceptably fat even though it is not acceptable to be fat at all. I will try and explain what seems a complicated paradox. Maureen and Anne are fairly typical of the women of their size who wrote or spoke to me about their feelings. They represent the woman who is definitely overweight by social and medical norms — somewhere between ten and a half and thirteen stones (150-180 lb). Their dress size is around 18-20, their height from about 5′2″ to 5′7″. All of these women have been made to feel abnormal or ugly by external pressures to conform to the perfect media-created image. They are unhappy because they feel abnormal — outsiders. And they blame themselves because they do not seem to be able to achieve the size and shape they 'should' be. Enter the concept of failure.

Yet examining these women's lives closely, they do not appear to have suffered *undue* harassment at the hands of doctors though they have certainly had their share of criticism. At their size, clothes are not a major problem, especially as the fashion industry is now paying lip-service to the fact that over half the women in Britain are a size 16 or over. Chain stores like Marks and Spencer stock clothes in sizes 18 and 20 and many clothes catalogues include these sizes in their normal range. Maureen, Anne and those of a similar size say they have not encountered discrimination or been the victims of direct prejudice though they feel its existence keenly. What they fear is the likelihood of such occurrences, having witnessed them in other women.

They are largely very active. Maureen swims, cycles, plays tennis and says it makes her wonder how she manages to be so fat. These women hate communal changing rooms, swimming pools and the beach. But they have not got to the point where they are housebound with fear and shame. They can manage turnstiles without the ignominy of getting wedged. They are not so likely to break chairs or find that the safety belts in planes and cars will not fasten.

Many fat women who wrote to me told me that they suffered some degree of agoraphobia, and in fact reports suggest that the incidence of agoraphobia is unusually high in fat people. Agoraphobia is usually an irrational fear of going out, irrational in the sense that there is not a known cause. But fat women express a fear of going out for reasons that they can name. The stress caused by being lectured, called names and patronised often by total strangers can prove too much and they retreat into the safety of their homes. This can then turn into a phobic fear of going outside. Sometimes this can spring from a single incident which may damage a woman's already vulnerable psyche and tip her over the edge into agoraphobia.

Jackie, a sixty-year-old extrovert who weighs twelve stones (168 lb), summed it up for her weight group:

No, there aren't any situations where I feel I stand out *enormously*. My doctor grumbles on and tries to put me on diets, but I ignore them. On the other hand she does not tell me that I am at risk of terrible things happening to me because of my weight. I once caught a glimpse of my notes at a hospital visit. The consultant had written: 'Mrs M is a plump, cheerful lady'. I rather liked that. I can fit into hospital gowns and cinema seats, even though they might not be as comfortable as I would like. I like wearing trousers and tops and don't have problems getting clothes that fit. I suppose the whole point is that although I am noticeably different from the slim, so-called normal sizes, I am not outstandingly, conspicuously different.

So society allows a little leeway for the moderately fat. But their response to me showed that their self-image and the damage to their psyche was in some cases just as crippling as for those who are much fatter. They may gain a tiny measure of acceptance in *some* contexts, but the central essence of acceptability remains the same. They are not slim. They are still 'the fatties'.

Eleanor Graham, the editor of the now sadly defunct magazine *Extra Special* is an elegant and beautiful middle-aged woman weighing eleven and a half stone (160 lb). She does not consider her weight a problem. But as she pointed out in one issue of the magazine,[3] Dusty Springfield, the immensely popular sixties pop-star making a comeback after 25 years of obscurity, was vilified by the *Sun*, which called her 'dumpy Springfield' and talked about her 'bulging figure' as 'bizarre' and her weight, which had 'ballooned', as 'staggering' and 'massive'. Eleanor pointed out in her editorial that Dusty weighed exactly the same as she did.

Unless we are the victims of blatant discrimination, or public figures like Dusty Springfield, we are unlikely to have our weight discussed in the public forum of the newspapers. But the attacks on those who moderately exceed the limits can be as destructive as those who are extremely fat. The resulting damage is the same. So Susan, who at twelve stones (168 lb), wrote to me of her deep unhappiness, described how her repeated attempts at dieting had failed consistently. She reached the point where a lifetime of being ostracised proved too much and she decided to take her own life. She bought a bottle of bleach at the chemists and: 'Only the sudden realisation that if I drank it as I intended to, they would have *won*, stopped me.'

So fat women, from ten stones (140 lb) to thirty stones (420 lbs) or more, handle their pain in a multitude of different ways, depending on their basic temperament, the degree of persecution they suffer and the amount of love they receive and, most importantly, received as children. In addition to that it must be remembered that fat women are also women without the adjective 'fat' and as such they are prey to all the other problems, feelings, disturbances, hormonal tempests — and joys — as every other woman. As well as coping with constant censure they are also saddled with popular concepts of the fat person's character. On the negative side are the familiar associations of fat with dim, dumb and dozy, as one woman put it — slow, stupid, ineffectual, incapable, inefficient, unintelligent, disabled and deformed.

The positive view of the fat person is only marginally easier to cope with. Fat people are happy and jolly, runs the myth, but this concurs with the metaphor of the tragic clown. On January 29, 1988, I took part in a programme with ex-Member of Parliament turned chat-show host Robert Kilroy-Silk which was sickeningly announced as 'The Fatties Fight Back'. I was intending to give rational, thought-provoking answers to his questions but instead I lost my temper. Why? Because the man asked that most inane of questions: 'Are fat people happy?' I gritted my teeth and asked *him* a few questions. What did he mean, I asked. You cannot generalise. Are thin people happy? Are people with GREY HAIR happy? I demanded of him, catching sight of his flop of silver hair. He was furious. After the programme he hissed at me: 'Why did you *do* that to me?' Not for nothing are television hospitality rooms dubbed 'hostility rooms'!

At the time when fatness was associated with prosperity and bounty, fertility and a cornucopia of good things, the concept of 'fat and happy' was an appropriate one. 'Laugh and grow fat' runs an old saying. Traditionally thin people were seen as miserable, ungenerous. Yet in spite of the seventy or so years of fat oppression, people of otherwise normal intelligence still persist with the notion that if you are fat, you will have a rounded, rosy-cheeked sort of personality.

THE COMPENSATING PERSONALITY:
THE JOKER

They cannot be blamed entirely for this misconception — though I am not saying that fat people are unhappy. I refuse to generalise. They are often very unhappy about being fat. The fat person has an outer and inner response to being the highly visible butt of jokes, sneers and pointing fingers. The outer response takes one of two forms. Either the fat woman withdraws from mainstream society, feeling unable to mix with her thin peers on equal terms, or develops the agoraphobic dislike of going out I mentioned before and simply becomes afraid to risk the hundreds of situations that will draw attention to her size. Or she develops what the psychologists call a compensating personality. This can operate in two ways and most people employ a combination of both, not usually consciously unless they have a fair degree of self-awareness.

The first ploy might be to distract the observer's attention away from the fat itself. This is often done by hiding in vast clothes which confer a kind of anonymity of body. Or dress might be bold, and by some people's standards, outrageous. While clothing provides the outward and visible message, it is the development of personality itself which is the real mechanism by which the fat woman distracts.

I well remember the beginnings of my own compensating personality. On my first day at high school, aged eleven, I was sitting with the rest of my new form, clad only in a vest and navy serge knickers, waiting to be measured for our gym uniform. I looked along the row of slightly-built girls and realised — I think for the first time in my life — that I didn't fit in. I was fat, and suddenly I was filled with panic. What was more I wore National Health specs with wire frames. I remember turning to the girl next to me, desperately needing reassurance. I can still see her clearly, placid looking, earnest, kind-faced. 'I'm fat,' I said to her miserably. 'And no one else is.' She looked at my hot-faced shame with sympathy and cast around for something nice to say. But she was an honest girl and she could not deny the truth of my outburst. 'Well,' she said, doubtfully, after a long pause for thought. 'You've got nice feet.'!

It did not get any better. The virago of a games teacher was moving down the row, embarrassingly measuring our chests for Aertex gym shirts. Everyone seemed to be a size 30 inches except for a couple of waif-like 28s. My turn came — and more burning shame. Not only was I fat, but I had breasts; 'you *are* a big girl'. And she called out my measurement so that everyone heard. I measured 36 inches. I very quickly learnt after that that being fat meant I started with a handicap, so to offset that I had to develop something extra in the way of personality if I was to be accepted as an equal. It was the start of the careful construction of the fat and happy persona, which I soon learned to project, thus misleading everyone about the real state of unhappiness underneath.

My schoolgirl defence was outrageous behaviour which ensured that I spent most evenings in detention and most of my school life being detested by the teachers for being a trouble-maker. That was a reasonable price to pay though for the admiration and acceptance of my peer group. I would accept any dare or challenge and became an outlet for their fantasies and the focus of their admiration. My real friends were my animals at home, amongst which I had four pet mice who enjoyed being kept in my pocket. I was dared one day to bring them to school and let them out when all was quiet in our Classics lesson — with the stuffiest teacher of them all. I did so, the other girls laughed, delighted at the commotion, yet safe from punishment while I ended up in the head's study as usual.

It was tiring, this compensating business. It required cunning and inventiveness and a constant watchfulness lest there be any cracks in the armour through which somebody might have glimpsed the pain. Games posed a problem at first. I could not run fast and I was naturally bad at aggressive field games like hockey, so there was danger there — of letting the side down. The only answer was distraction again, so I pretended that I was a pony, cantering along the side of the pitch in a dreamy fantasy world, snorting and head tossing while the others tore up and down the pitch. They forgave me for not participating, so great was their delight at witnessing my flouting of all the barked orders from the games teacher. That imaginary pony became part of my personality. When I could not cope with the harshness of constantly being in trouble in order to defend my reputation of living dangerously, I merged myself into my pony character so that 'they' could not reach into me.

Eating at school was difficult. The other girls assumed that because I was fat I would eat anything, and indeed I was often dreadfully hungry at school. We had an iniquitous and senseless rule in the dining room — when everyone had finished, the whole table had to put up their hands, and the teacher on duty would come and inspect plates to see that they were cleared of every mouthful before we were allowed to clear away. As we were not permitted to refuse a portion of anything when we queued up with our plates — and those dinner ladies had no mercy — it caused problems about food which we genuinely didn't like. My table put their trust in me. Give it to old dustbin, they said — and partly to oblige them and partly because I was sometimes hungry, I would accept their leavings and so clear the plates. It went wrong one day — we had a very sickly lemon curd pudding which no one liked, and I ended up with six helpings on my plate. Of course I couldn't finish it and the old hatchet face came to inspect. 'You will finish your pudding — every scrap of it,' she said threateningly and I can still recall the lurch of protest from my stomach. She stood over me, the rest of the table in thrall — and the inevitable happened — I was violently and ignominously sick all over the table. And had to clear it up.

I carried on being the joker, but inside I bled. The tears of the clown. I ate because I was unhappy about my size, and I was unhappy about my size because I was eating . . . But I continued to elicit gasps of horror from our rather old-fashioned teachers and was only saved from expulsion by a rather wise headmistress who discussed my behaviour with my mother and had more insight than most of her staff. Years later, when I had occasion to meet one or two of them on equal terms, I discovered that it had never occurred to them that my 'bad' behaviour was a symptom of distress and that I was caught in a cycle of unhappiness and comfort eating, completely ignorant of the fact that I might be liked for myself regardless of my brave deeds! But at the time it was too risky. The very nature of the fat person's compensating personality is an apology — I am an outcast, but if I offer you this or this to make up for my shortcomings, will you accept me?

The compensating personality is a treacherous thing. It served me well for most of my life, but it becomes something in you but not of you. And as years go by it becomes more and more difficult to distinguish between the real person and the layers, which have grown like an oyster shell round the vulnerable self.

Another variation on the joker is the fat person who constantly mocks herself in front of others. 'I'll never get through that gap,' she laughs, or 'Watch out, this chair might not take my weight. Bessie Bunter on the warpath.' Some people are quite unable to do this — I have always been one of them — but for others it is a way of getting in first, and staving off the inevitable digs. I have a very large friend who, in the middle of lunch with us at home, suddenly disappeared in a welter of splintering wood as her chair disintegrated. The family held their breath in case she was hurt, but when she had recovered from the immediate shock she was in there first with the joky remarks about no chair being safe with her and had we got any others we wanted demolished.

The incident was an extraordinary mixture of comedy and pathos, not to mention concern. Landing heavily, as she did on our quarry-tiled floor knocked her about considerably. Getting up quickly from my own place and going to the other side of the table, I saw my friend, sitting helplessly on her bottom, shocked, somewhat humiliated but determined to laugh. And the dreadful thing was that seeing her there, the chair in matchwood around her, the laughter rose up in me until it was uncontrollable and burst out. I, of all people was the one who identified with her, and was upset and feeling responsible, as you do if something happens in your house. But taking their cue from me, one by one the rest of the family dissolved into helpless laughter. Why, I do not know. I am sure that we would not have laughed had she not initially laughed at herself. I am also sure that in her position I would have cried with shame. I still cannot explain why it was so funny though I don't think it was to do with her weight. Rather with the sudden disappearance of someone who until that moment had been engrossed in her meal with the rest of us and then dispatched an entire chair. The nature of slapstick I suppose. But would we have laughed had it been a thin person? I hope so.

THE COMPENSATING PERSONALITY: THE NICE GIRL

Different aspects, then, of the entertainer persona. The other common compensating personality, which often combines with the first, is the nice girl. Again, the feeling is that it is necessary to have something extra to offer.

Because you have already stepped out of line by being fat, you must prove that for that sin you can make reparation by having an extra grace. So the woman compensating by being nice becomes everybody's friend, giving abundantly but never looking for any return. She tries to live up to the ancient symbolism of abundance, only it is abundance of herself, her qualities and her time that she offers so freely.

It does not take long to become enmeshed in the role for it carries powerful incentives, and the personality which seeks to compensate for its shortcomings will in turn look for compensations to act as balm on the wounds of others' rejection. So for every unkind remark, every humiliating experience concerning her size there will be a balancing reward as someone seeks her out for her particular kind of friendship, or warmth or help.

Long before I was twenty I gained a reputation for being someone boys could talk to about their problems. I resented it — who wouldn't when they are still in their teens! — but I did not dare repudiate this role because I realised I might be left with nothing. Later, when I took a course in journalism at college, I hovered on a brink between continuing to be the warm-hearted Earth Mother, to whom boys could confide their problems, and retreating altogether into a natural shyness and feeling of isolation because of being 'different'. I chose to stay in circulation.

I did marry, very young, in fact, and to a very thin man — one of the 'seven-stone weaklings'! I worked in the media where pressure to conform is probably greater than anywhere else but by that time I had a well-rounded persona. I never got rattled, and I was *never* unpleasant or short-tempered with anyone. And I continued to add layers to my personality in order to become acceptable. When I spent some years at home after the births of my children, I was the one friends came to, to talk things over. My kitchen was always full of women drinking tea! And later, back at work at the BBC I became even more of a mother figure, partly because I was older and had children I suppose. Tormented, tortured love affairs were always being sorted out in my office.

I'm not saying I resented this. It met the need to be needed which is part of the human condition and it is very flattering to hear things like 'I've never told anyone else this but I feel I can tell you' and 'I can talk to you about anything'.

But there came a time when I was working hard, looking after my family and seemed to have an enormous number of people still drinking tea round my table and weeping metaphorically or otherwise on my shoulder. My lame ducks, my mother always called them. And they began to be too much for me. I did not have the energy to spare. I began to dread the phone ringing and those words 'Can I come and talk to you?' I was becoming drained and yet did not dare say so, for I did not value myself enough to believe that I could be wanted as a friend without providing this extra service.

The pressure built up over the years because it was always one-way traffic. People associated my large bulk with serenity and assumed I had no problems of my own. Time after time I would hear them express envy that I was 'so placid' and that 'nothing ever got on top of me'. This often included remarks about my size, harsh, stabbing comments that were never meant or perceived as such but carried the assumption that what mattered to 'normal' women did not apply to me, as though being very fat had something to do with being beyond normal feelings and therefore not minding. So friends struggling with their extra half a stone would say, 'I wish I could be like you. It must be wonderful not to care.'

The first signs of the persona cracking came when a friend came over and I was depressed. She was almost outraged. She actually said that she could not cope with me being depressed because she always relied on me being the same and comforting her when *she* was low. She made it clear that she had never seen it as a reciprocal relationship in that sense. It was a time of crisis; I felt I was being pulled apart.

The cracks extended to me responding to remarks made about my size. I told my friends that I *did* mind, and several were offended. For years they had taken their cues from the image of me that I had given them. I had worked so hard to hide the pain of being outcast that I found it difficult to differentiate what was really me and what was the public face. It took therapy to sort that out and it still feels scary to allow myself to express the same needs, rights and feelings as those of normal weight.

I have used this example of my own years of constructing a compensating personality because it is the one I know best. I now understand how it comes about and how many of us do the same thing. It is about not permitting ourselves to be real, because we are in a constant state of apology and penance. We want society to overlook and forgive our 'failing', whether it is perceived as deliberate and calculated gluttony and sloth, or whether as lack of will-power, self-discipline and self-respect. One state is active, one passive but it makes no difference to the evaluation made of us. We have failed. We respond like naughty, contrite children: 'If I am good — if I do the washing-up, tidy my room, chop the wood — will you approve of me and love me?' But only children who have cause for feeling insecure need to earn love and approval in this way. The happy child is the one who feels she can be 'naughty' — not with impunity but with freedom.

The result of constant stigmatization and negative evaluation is that those who are the target of these pressures come to believe they are responsible for their state and so they create a self-fulfilling prophecy. As one woman wrote:

Recently my husband showed some family photos to his colleagues at work. When I next phoned him at work I was answered by a man I had not met. He said 'Now I've seen a photo of you I understand why your husband spends so much time at the office.' I laughed and joked; 'Yes, not a pretty sight.' But I was heartbroken, have cried so much and lost all confidence since then.

It is all too easy to believe that we are the cause of a great deal of trouble to others by wanting to exist as fat people in the same society as those who keep the rules of normality. We may create disruption as we tread on people's feet, trying to make our way to a theatre seat in the centre of the row. Or we may be made to feel guilty and distressed at the harm we are told we are doing to our children by being deviant and by leaving them to bear the brunt of jibes about their fat mothers from their school-fellows. The emphasis is always placed on the effect our weight has on others. I have never heard anyone talk about how dreadful it must be to be the focus of all eyes as one tries to manoeuvre a fat body through a forest of legs and knees in a space hardly big enough for a cat. Because it is not an easy thing to do, there are plenty of thin people who bump people and tread on their toes, but there is an acceptance that this does happen in such ridiculously narrow spaces and a word of apology usually brings an understanding smile from all but the most short-tempered individuals. If you are thin it is the fault of the theatre, packing the rows too close behind each other. If you are fat, then you are taking up more than your share of space — you have transgressed, yet again.

The fat mother does not *need* telling that she is a source of embarrassment to her child. But what of the understanding shown to her? Not only does she have to cope with society's onslaught on her own behalf, she is fully aware of her child's predicament. In her guilt she colludes with those who condemn her for tainting her child's school and social life with the results of her deviance. She is inclined to believe that she may be damaging her child.

I bought a book called *The Divine Supermarket –* *Shopping for God in America*. This has nothing at all to do with weight — I was interested in it because it explores the phenomenon of America's diversity of religious denominations, sects and cults. However, I could not get beyond page 15, where the author (who is English, Eton educated) begins his journey in a hired recreational vehicle or RV: 'I was happy with the camper. It handled more like an ordinary car than I had expected . . . I felt quite gleeful when passing trucks or other RVs — fat, complacent overweight vehicles, much I surmised, like their occupants. I had become obsessed with Obese Persons, who seemed to be everywhere, in and around New York, blocking supermarket checkouts, blocking escalators, elbowing one off sidewalks. They seemed to be constantly munching, licking, sucking, masticating: I felt no twinge of compassion for their offensive corpulence, only disgust at their ugliness and lack of self-restraint.'

The stigmatization of the overweight is unyielding and uncompromising. Imagine the utopian scenario if, in the theatre situation for example, the collusion were with the fat person seeking her seat and the condemnation reserved for theatre managements who, through their greed in squeezing so many people in, made unrealistic demands of the human body. How differently the fat mother would feel if parents taught their children that bodies came in all different sizes and shapes and that every one of them is equally acceptable, and if teachers and social workers did not disguise their own contempt with concern for the child — because in this utopian state there would be no contempt to disguise. Even without utopian expectations, why do we teach our children to be so judgemental? Prejudice, discrimination, contempt, stigmatization and rejection are not only sadistic, fascist and intensely painful for fat people. These things have a serious effect on physical, mental and emotional health; an effect which is real, and must not be trivialised. In addition, the fat person bears this alone. Although, in America, we have the wonderful solidarity of NAAFA, we have no laws to protect us from fattism, no Size Relations Board, no equal opportunities watchdogs. Thin supremacy reigns as white supremacy once did. One woman said to me: 'I'm fat and I'm black. And I know which is worse. Being fat in your culture.'

STRESS

When we are confronted with the hundreds, thousands of embarrassing, humiliating and isolating situations that our society chooses to visit upon us because of our size, most of us react with stress. Every time we go hot, feel ourselves breaking out in a cold sweat, find our hearts racing and wish the ground would open and swallow us up, our body is reacting with stress. Our adrenalin is constantly being called into action, flooding our bodies with hormones which were designed to be dispersed by the primitive fight or flight mechanism. For a fat person this can happen several times a day — in fact it often becomes such a familiar part of her response to the world that she does not notice the instances of stress as she would if confronted by a large fierce dog or footsteps quickening behind her on a dark night. In those situations she is aware in some part of her that she may have to take aggressive or evasive action and in that way she externalizes the focus of the stress. Unless we are able to get angry — and express the anger — with the doctor who says we cannot be helped unless we lose weight, the schoolboy who jeers 'fat frump' as we walk past, or the snooty shop assistant who says with distaste: '*Not* in *your* size' — then we swallow and internalize our stressful responses, usually offering a placatory one in its place as our compensating personality has conditioned us to do.

In addition to the myriad instances, major or minor, that may affect us during the course of any one day, fat women carry a constant burden of tension, largely unrecognized because it is always there, underlying everything we do or feel. It is our unconscious, watchful response to the injuries we have suffered, for some people over most of their lives. It is the part that is on guard the whole time so that we will not be caught out by chance remarks, the apparent concern of our friends, the fat jokes on television. It is the part of us that reacts when we read in the newspapers that a celebrity has died of a heart attack, going to town on her weight and leaving us in no doubt that we might meet the same fate. It is our response to the bombardment of media pressure that tells us we must look good, which means being thin, and medical pressure from all quarters that threatens us with sudden death and shortened lives. Stress means the despairing tightrope we walk between our desire and willingness to become slim and free ourselves from these threats and our inability to do so because diets do not work; not to mention our anger that we cannot be left to choose the way we want to be. If we have children there is no shortage of reminders that we may not live to see them grow up or to enjoy our grandchildren, or even to enjoy our biblical three score years and ten. Stress is what makes us wake in the middle of the night, when everything is at its most bleak, and become convinced that the pain we feel is not the indigestion we thought it was at supper time, it is finally the dreaded fatal heart attack we have been warned about; and as we lie there, paralysed with fear, we wonder what death will be like and if there is anything after it, and how will our children manage without us.

Does that sound dramatic? Maybe, but it is a scenario drawn from the fears and feelings of a host of fat women, all of whom have experienced some or all of this degree of stress. And have had the additional stress of hiding it, not being able to confide for fear of being thought neurotic, even to their nearest. When I advertised in the *Guardian* for people to write to me about their feelings and experiences of being fat, I found that many letters started or finished with variations of the words: 'This is the first time I have really explained to anyone what I feel like about being fat'. *Over*-dramatic? Certainly not. It must be remembered that there are very few situations or very few people who will affirm the fat woman's identity — *as* a fat woman — socially or medically. I have found that even the least judgemental, most understanding people will say gently: 'But wouldn't you feel better if you were slim/thinner/if you lost just a bit of weight? In other words, when you cease to *be* and concentrate on *becoming*. That is isolation and it is extreme stress.

In 1986 I became part of the team producing a new women's magazine. *Extra Special* was the first of its kind in Britain: specifically for large women. Fat women. Its message was clear and unequivocal. We told our readers: You have the right to be large, as large as you want to be, as large as you are. At the launch party for the magazine I found that I was feeling unusually free and confident and also something much less definable, a kind of lightness as though some nagging worry had been lifted. I did not realize until half way through the evening that this was because the only reason I was *there* was because I was fat, that I was not presenting my personal and professional qualities along with an unspoken apology for my body.

And that my body was like that of everyone else who was involved in the launch. The same thing happened a few weeks later when Independent Television ran a programme about fat women. All of us taking part were very large indeed. ITV put us up in the Holiday Inn where we had dinner together and swam in their beautiful heated pool. We enjoyed our dinner with no one tutting or watching how much we ate, we met at the pool and swam without fear of getting 'those looks' when we appeared in swimsuits. And we shared a tremendously valuable solidarity, a sense of feeling good about ourselves, even to the extent of perceiving the programme presenter, a size 12, as rather scrawny! I mention these incidents because they are the only occasions I can think of when the undermining, ever-present stress of being outcast was *gone,* really completely gone, and I felt utterly, entirely myself. It made me see how different I would be if I could experience that unity and acceptance more often. It is quite different from those friends who love you for what you are, and genuinely do so, but could not bear to be like you. However much someone thinks of you, it is undermining to know that they would not want to look like you.

That freedom from stress, though short-lived, made me acutely aware of physical, mental and emotional differences in me. The sense of physical relaxation was marvellous — just walking into the hotel dining room was a liberating experience, knowing that it did not matter at all what the other diners thought because I was with a supportive group of women who were all like me. I found I did not have that tense, waiting-to-be-pounced-on tautness that usually accompanies me when walking through any kind of public place. Mentally and physically I knew perfect peace because I was accepted. It really is simple.

I have not found that kind of relief from stress in slimming clubs because they are not about acceptance. The solidarity there is that of a group of women committed to changing themselves — it is achievement oriented and with elements of competitiveness, success and failure. Stress thrives in those conditions — and I am not saying that some kinds of stress are necessarily always a bad thing. They can give the impetus to a goal, but the desire to reach that goal has to be there first. Slimming clubs have a unity of purpose but approval is conditional and certain types of personality go under, rather than respond in competitive situations. If that ethos does not strike a stirring chord but rather fills you with dread, then slimming clubs will just be another source of pressure. Besides, they do not offer a way to lose weight permanently and they are ridiculously expensive.

A local store had a day in aid of the British Heart Foundation. Helpful looking women stood around waiting to answer questions and a table contained a pile of booklets about the heart. They terrified me. Being fat means being conditioned to the medical equivalent of horror stories. It is simply too scary to read them. It is not even helpful because we cannot put into practice their message when we know that 98 per cent of weight loss is regained and that the dangers of losing and regaining are greater than of either losing *or* gaining. Not that the British Heart Foundation sets out to petrify us in its literature, merely to warn. But what of other 'experts'?

> Fat, obese, overweight, tubby, portly, corpulent, rotund. Call yourself anything you want. You know what you are. It bothers you. It depresses you. And it should frighten you. You've been warned, time and time again, what that oppressive extra burden could mean to your health — high blood pressure, heart attack, diabetes . . . early death.[4]

So we have the physicians — humanity's helpmeets — on the one hand *frightening* us to death and on the other admitting that there is no remedy for our condition, while continuing to blame us for not doing something about it.

I am not using a mere colloquialism when I say 'frightening us to death'. There is an increasing body of enlightened medical opinion which maintains that if fat people do suffer a greater than average incidence of life-threatening heart disease and high blood pressure then these conditions are more likely to be caused by the stress of being frightened, threatened and stigmatised than the obesity itself.

The way to combat this is to look at the historical and cultural facts. In societies which value fatness, and revere and celebrate large bodies, those people do not develop the so-called obesity-related diseases and life-threatening conditions. And in periods of history — and that includes our own Western history — where thinness was considered a sign of poor health and lack of strength, and fatness was seen as wonderfully healthy, what happened? The thin died young and the fat lived to a ripe old age.

Hilde Bruch and Llewellyn Louderback have both made extensive studies of the cultural history of weight and health, and (separately) they arrived at these conclusions:

It is my personal conviction that this hostile attack on weight as a shameful evil has contributed to a large extent to making overweight and obesity such serious health problems . . . there is no doubt about the damaging effect on mental health of the current campaign against overweight. *Hilde Bruch*

The fat, who are kept from developing their fullest capacity as human beings and whose links joining them to other human beings and to the world around them are weaker, are denied the deeper roots of the will to live, are denied the elementary psychological safeguards against illness and premature death. Our constant harping on the spurious issue of health seals their doom, for since we expect them to fall apart at an earlier age than other people, many of them obligingly do so. *Llewellyn Louderback*[5]

I do not want fat people reading this to be alarmed at the above prognosis. I would not have included it if I did not believe, and have evidence, that it can be defused and reversed. What in effect has happened is that we have had a spell put on us, a curse. It is similar to the practices of certain tribal societies where those with power and influence put a curse on some unfortunate who has crossed them. 'You will die' they say — and these people do, because they believe it. It is time for us to disempower the curse (see Chapter 8).

At Manchester University, Cary Cooper and his team have done in-depth research into stress in all its forms. Professor Cooper has the chair of Organisational Psychology at the University of Manchester Institute of Science and Technology (UMIST). Cooper's verdict on stress is that for the fat person it is the real bugbear, a very real problem which cannot be ignored. Being fat forces a person into certain roles that are not constitutionally right for them for the reasons already discussed — namely, that they are having to play parts to placate or compensate and that they live under constant attack. Stress itself is the component of the risk to the cardiovascular system: 90 per cent of all heart attacks are caused by arterial problems. The biochemistry of stress causes noradrenalin to be pumped round our bodies and this hormone damages the walls of the coronary arteries. The body then has to produce fibrinogen, a clotting substance, to patch up the damaged parts of these arteries and in doing so causes them to narrow.[6]

Diet is also important for arteries and there cannot be many still unaware of the importance of avoiding artery-clogging saturated fats. A high-fat diet combined with intense stress shoots up the risk of heart disease or attack, but correct the diet and remove the stress and the fat person is at no greater risk, or only marginally so, than anyone else. The key there is the removal of the stress which is culturally created in the West.

Dr Margaret Mackenzie is an anthropologist who has made a speciality of studying body image in different cultures. In Western Samoa she discovered that women gain weight after each pregnancy until they become very large indeed. In that culture the fat body is seen as desirable and admirable, especially in middle age when the women are permitted to perform the dances frequently commented upon by visitors to the Pacific. They move and dance freely without restraint or shame because there is no stigma attached to their body size.

Yet these fat women do not suffer from heart disease or high blood pressure. Even when they cross cultures and migrate to America only three out of a hundred women who weighed more than two hundred pounds showed any signs of hypertension. Margaret Mackenzie's findings among the Samoan women have led her to postulate that the root cause of the so-called fat related diseases may well have nothing to do with the strain put on the body by weight but with the damage done by being in an almost constant state of alarm and stress. [7]

American biomedical researcher, Dr Paul Ernsberger cites a study which found that 81 per cent of the world's cultures consider overall plumpness or moderate fatness to be desirable for females, and fat hips or thighs are considered attractive in 90 per cent of all cultures. The thinnest ethnic group are Oriental peoples and Western Europeans, particularly the English and French.

The fattest ethnic groups are those who endured centuries of starvation — American Indians, Jews, Poles, other East Europeans, blacks and Hispanics. Britain has had stable food supplies for centuries. So it is here that we find the tasteless and bizarre juxtaposition photographed by Mike Wells in a Fulham Street. Two advertising hoardings hang side by side on a wall. One is an advertisement for sheer tights, showing a pair of thin legs and captioned: 'Legs that men dream about'. The other also depicts a thin pair of legs; it is for Christian Aid Week and the caption pleads: 'Help those left behind in the human race'.[8] It is an image that places thinness firmly in context.

Studies done among even the very fat in cultures where it is considered normal do not show decreased life expectancy. Some show a greater life expectancy for the very fat (for more detail about this, see Chapter 7). They do not have heart disease and increased blood pressure because they are free from the dual stress of persecution and dieting.

They celebrate their fat. A friend told me about the very large women she saw when she was living in Mozambique. They wore tight, short skirts, she said, to show off their bodies, and took pity on her slimness. Another friend had a holiday in Tonga for which she had spent months getting her figure 'in trim' with diet and exercise and good strong doses of self-discipline. She had looked forward to lying on sunkissed beaches, exposing her beaten-into-shape body. She was disappointed. Among the huge black Tongan people she was as insignificant as a stick insect. And for Tongan men she had as much sex appeal as one.

When people from fat-loving cultures migrate to America or some European countries they respond either by being driven to lose weight in order to conform with their new found society or by showing amazement at what they consider to be our topsy-turvy ideals. I shall never forget talking to a West Indian woman who had been living in Britain for some ten years and was still feeling bemused at our obsession with thinness: 'Why do you English women put up with those terrible clothes for fat women?' she asked me. Why indeed? And then she told me how she had passed a shop window on her way to work every day where there was displayed the most gorgeous dress. 'I went into the shop,' she said. 'But it was just as I feared. It only went up to size 16. What use is that to anyone?' She continued to hanker after the frock and being a positive thinker she soon had a brainwave. She went and bought *two* size 16s and made them into one dress.

I received a letter from an African woman, at university in England, showing a very different cultural approach to fat — a reversal of the Western attitude and a powerful illustration of different notions of acceptability:

I've always been much taller than average and extremely slender. In my part of Africa the ideal woman is large, big-busted, big-bottomed. I was made to feel extremely miserable during my teenage years, especially at school, for being the direct opposite of what was considered to be attractive.

I've been in Britain ten months now and I'm still not used to the way people enthuse over my slim figure. Or to the continual pressures on the female population, mainly through the media, to make themselves into human matchsticks. Why should one type be better than another? We all have different physiques due to hereditary and other factors, surely all that matters is that we should be reasonably healthy?

Perhaps it is only by looking at the appreciation of the large female body in other cultures that we may be able to get a sense of perspective and proportion. The previously mentioned juxtaposition of the advertisement hoardings both featuring thin legs suggests to me that our Western preoccupation with thinness is a sickness and a direct historical result of never being deprived of staple foods. There is also a class factor in operation here; studies have shown that fatness is almost exclusively confined to the lower and middle classes and indeed it is not difficult to see this in action. It is rare to see anything more than a slight degree of plumpness amongst upper class and upwardly mobile women which may explain the excessive media criticism of any member of the royal family who exceeds a size 12. Paul Ernsberger has a theory that better standards of living for the working classes in the early part of the twentieth century allowed them to become stout for the first time, whereas in Victorian and Edwardian times, corpulence was a symbol of wealth and status. In order to create a visible difference between the working classes and themselves, the upper class elite of the early 20th century took slimness as a definition for their status, and still do.[9]

The merging of cultures which is giving us the Global Village concept is a source of problems for ethnic societies attempting to take on Western values. In the Italian/American community of Roseto in Pennsylvania, fatness was normal and the heart attack rate was negligible. The Rosetans lived as a largely enclosed community, conserving their Italian culture and eating habits — by American definition they ate all the 'wrong' foods. They were healthy and lived for a long time, confounding the perceived nutritional wisdom of the time. During the 1960s the people of Roseto became more Americanized; one of the telling signs of change was the opening of a Weight Watchers group in the town. By the 1970s the heart attack rate was the same as everywhere else in Pennsylvania.[10]

Kim Chernin talks of a woman she counselled for an eating disorder, a woman who was slender 'with that gaunt, fashionable slenderness so popular today but not natural to her'. The woman, Anita, had been in therapy for fifteen years. She induced herself to vomit four times a day, every day. Anita came from Panama, migrating to America when she was fourteen with several members of her family. Straightaway the women went and enrolled in diet groups. Her mother put her on a diet. She was taking after her mother —

> a big woman, but now we thought it was fat. And all this was part of the way she was preparing me to become an American, to take part in this society. I can't blame her. She wanted me to be a typical American girl. And that meant slender. And that meant diet. And that meant not cook or eat the way we ate in Panama.

This change of cultural definition led to a painful split between Anita and her mother. She became a gymnast, a long distance runner, a skier, and kept herself awake to study at night by taking diet pills — amphetamines. But then the years of driving herself caught up with her:

> I started to lie around in bed and eat . . . here I was, the fruit of all this discipline and hectoring and training, my family's pride, their ticket to the new world, a walking talking American doll, a bit too tall, but just-right slender and now I lay in bed and ate bagsfull of doughnuts, dozens of them, jelly-filled. And when I thought I'd burst from eating, and was terrified I wouldn't be able to stand up the next day and go back to the job, I went over to the toilet and taught myself how to vomit . . . That wasn't an eating disorder. That was my life cracking apart. It was practically suicide.[11]

Anthropologist Margaret Mackenzie talks of 'A new US export — fear of fat'. She describes a visit to the island of

Rarotonga in Polynesia, summoned by an anxious nurse who was caring for a baby she believed to be seriously underweight but who was pronounced as normal by the visiting nutritionist whose purpose was to educate the people about the dangers of obesity. Mackenzie describes the method as having 'well-intentioned but punitive strategies, evident in the denial of new uniforms to a category of (fat) health professionals intended to be exemplars of the latest medical knowledge to the general population'. The obesity campaign had started because of a survey of weight and blood pressure in adults in 1983. The senior public health nurse confessed to Mackenzie that she was feeling guilty — she had just eaten an ice-cream. Margaret Mackenzie is not opposed to the idea of introducing good nutrition but she sees the negative and harmful effects of the fat prejudice, already implicit in restricting uniforms and condemning people to wear tattered clothes until they became thin. Lives *may* be saved, she says, but the ramifications of the methods used are likely to undermine the dignity of the Pacific islanders by introducing the new notions of prejudice and failure. Worse, they may cause a series of diseases associated with fear of fatness.

Before she left, Mackenzie met another friend for a drink — because she refused to eat anything. Most of the conversation was about her friend's weight, how fat, ugly, ungainly and ashamed she felt. No matter how hard she tried to diet, she found herself at times voraciously hungry, eating the food she was trying to avoid and hating herself for doing so. Mackenzie says: 'My beautiful, graceful friend has already succumbed to an eating disorder.'[12]

In February 1989 two British nutritionists were sent to Tonga by Voluntary Service Overseas with a view to educating the islanders in good nutrition. The intention was to reach those at risk from cardio-vascular disease and those who are seriously overweight. In a written statement, the VSO says that the Tongan problem is due to the fact that the people are moving away from their traditional healthy island diet of roots, fruit, seafood and meat and are importing foodstuffs which are nutritionally worthless and with high levels of fat. This is contributing to the island's increasing problems of overweight, diabetes, high blood pressure, heart disease, dental caries and gout.

While it is true that a Westernised junk-food diet will certainly cause many of the diseases mentioned, I am disturbed at the emphasis on treating overweight Tongans. This can only mean putting them on a diet while the need would appear to be to re-educate them about a *healthy* way of eating. The tragedy is that so many rich and colourful cultures see themselves as anachronistic and long for the shoddiness — which to them appears glamorous — of the Western lifestyle.

> You weigh your self-worth on the bathroom scale.
>
> Martha Zinger, clinical psychologist who organized the demonstration against dieting in Huntington, WV, where crowds of women publicly smashed up bathroom scales.

I read a delightful anecdote of the way an African public health poster, designed with the intention of counteracting the prevailing positive images of fat, backfired. The poster showed a fat woman and an overloaded lorry with a flat tyre; the caption read 'Both carry too much weight'. People not only thought the woman was wonderfully fat, but also assumed she was rich, since she had a lorry weighed down with her possessions. A true case of *mens sana in corpore sano*. [13]

SELF-IMAGE

The animal kingdom rejects as hostile any member of its own species that differs considerably from the norm. The outsider is literally driven out of the fold or the pack. Think, on a simplistic level, of the story of the Ugly Duckling and you have it. It was not so much that he was ugly as that he was not like the rest of the brood.

> We've been conditioned to find overweight people unattractive and we attach words like 'greedy' and 'overindulgent' to them. But some indulgences seem to be allowed while others aren't. The lad from the rugby team who drinks 12 pints of beer is not considered greedy in the same way as the woman who eats a whole packet of biscuits in an evening.
>
> Cosmopolitan, September 1993

Fat people are abnormal by the simple, unemotive factual definition of the word, which is not conforming to type. Type is laid down by the way a culture develops and it responds to such stimuli as wealth or lack of it, materialism and external trend-setting influences: fashion and media. Another potent factor, especially since the years of the Thatcher government in Britain is the emphasis on achievement and goal-orientation. And in that is contained all the twentieth century's ideals surrounding the work ethic; self-discipline, self-control, asceticism. Fear of failure is now one of the most important motivators and some experts on the anorexic personality believe this is directly responsible for the sharp rise in anorexia in the last decade or so. The pressure to succeed in college, school, university and employment proves too much for many young people so they demonstrate their powers of achievement in the only way they can — by starving themselves and producing the visible result of a perfectly self-disciplined body.[14]

Obviously in such a culture it should follow that greed is highly unacceptable. And yet this is not so. We are more materialist and consumerist than ever before. We are exhorted to go for the top, to be acquisitive, to buy our own homes, have the holidays we want, the best (private) medical care and education. Technology tempts us on all sides with its armoury of domestic gadgetry so that now we do not even get up from our chair to adjust the television, we do it with a remote control.

I am sickened at the price paid for a meal in a restaurant whenever I go out for a professional lunch. But this is run of the mill — it is not seen as greed. If I chose the most expensive low calorie dishes on the menu, that would meet with more social approval than if I opted for cheaper, more plentiful or 'fattening' food. *That* in a fat person would be regarded as greed.

Women are regarded as the givers and feeders, embodying self-sacrifice. The image of the 'good family' is that of a slim, well-groomed mother, self-effacingly eating small portions, while men and large, bonny, robust boys are urged to 'tuck in' — they deserve a good meal after that hard day at work or expending all that energy playing football. So deeply is this ingrained that many mothers automatically give their families the biggest and best pieces of meat, the crispiest roast potatoes and plenty of them.

This is another reason why it is so much more unacceptable for a woman to be fat. She has not remained in her defined role. She shows visible proof of 'having had too much'. She has fed herself, perhaps while others go without. I have an extremely well-adjusted fat friend who suffered none of these dilemmas. When her family were small, she served herself first:

Look, I went to a lot of trouble keeping house and cooking for that lot. And what did they do? Sat around and waited for meals to be served to them. I didn't mind that, I accepted it as my role. But I felt that having toiled over the preparation and cooking of a meal I should have some reward. So I served myself with the biggest or the most succulent piece of meat, and all the vegetables I wanted. And if there was anything special going — peaches, for example — I kept them as treats for myself. Why not? Their turn would come when they grew up and started slaving themselves.

My immediate response to this was shock-horror, what selfishness, it is our duty as women and as mothers to nurture, to deny ourselves. But this woman is one of the very few who genuinely has no problems with self-esteem or self-image. She values herself and does not see that being fat means that she should value herself less. And of course she is right. Is there a connection between her self-nurturing attitude and her positive self-image?

Dr Jill Welbourne, a psychiatrist at the Bristol Royal Infirmary who specialises in eating disorders, feels very strongly that women must break through the myth that it is somehow self-indulgent to feed oneself as well as we do others: 'Why do we feel that if we are having people to supper we must cook something special, perhaps with a nice sauce and a pudding when we wouldn't dream of doing that for ourselves?'

There is something irrefutably logical about Jill Welbourne's argument. She herself is a big woman, tall and fat by our received standards. But she has a positive self-image which makes her extremely successful in her work with patients who have disturbed body images. She tells a story which neatly illustrates her philosophy:

I was cooking my supper one night when I was at medical school. I had a lamb chop waiting to go in, some nice vegetables and I was in the middle of making an onion sauce when my room mate came in. 'I didn't know you were having anyone for supper', she said. I told her I wasn't. She said: 'You can't mean you're doing all that — going to all that trouble just for yourself?' WHO BETTER! I said to her.

This is the difference between loving and hating our bodies. The pleasures of eating good food have given way to a different kind of gratification — the acquisition of material possessions and the craving for status — the fruits of Thatcherism in Britain. We are encouraged to value *things* above people, to judge people by what they own, or have achieved, rather than for what they *are*.

Janette is a freelance editor with a husband and one daughter. Their combined salary in 1992 was £80,000 gross. They have a large country house, a cottage in Dorset and a villa abroad. They eat in restaurants most of the time because they can afford to. Janette wears expensive clothes and is a regular visitor to health farms and beauty salons. She has her hair done once a week and the family has three exotic foreign holidays a year. She admits that she loves going shopping just for the sheer pleasure of spending money and bringing home new things, most of which she does not need. The only real blight on her life is her weight. At 5'7", Janette weighs nine and a half stones (133 lb). Not overweight by the most severe definition. But she pinches imaginary rolls of flesh and moans about the cellulite on her thighs. She wants to be eight stones (112 lb). Her body has not allowed her to diet to eight stones as that is far too low for it and fortunately she does not have an anorexic personality. So when she tries to diet, she very soon starts eating more and craves cakes and chocolate. She thinks she is 'fat' because she eats too much. She sees herself as undisciplined because she has not stuck to her diets. For her it is always a case of 'One day I *will* do it . . .'

Janette was prepared to be totally open and honest about her feelings when I told her I was writing a book about fat women. She disagrees absolutely with the messages contained in the book. She said to me:

Look, you seem like a nice person and you're intelligent. You've got quite good skin and hair. I can't understand how you can bear to go around being as fat as you are. I'd rather die! Have you been to Weight Watchers? Think how much better you'd feel, and look, if you were slim. Think of the clothes you could wear. It would be a whole new life opening up to you. Doesn't it *worry* you? Why do you think you eat too much?

I told her that I would welcome everything she had to say on the subject of fat, because it would be good to have a real person's feelings about it alongside all the research and collective evidence. I said she could be as insulting as she liked as it would make good copy for me. She continued:

The reason I don't want to be fat is because fat people are hated. They are usually sloppy and lazy, they have no will-power or self-respect. If they did they would diet and become slim. They don't care enough about the way they look and I never really think of them as belonging with the rest of us. I know this sounds like prejudice, but you did ask me to be honest. I would respect you a lot more if you told me you were going to write a book to encourage fat people to diet so that they could have more of a place in society. You don't have to be fat. If I didn't watch what I ate, I could creep right up to ten or eleven stones. And — I just don't like looking at fat people. I find all those rolls and bulges revolting and those round moon faces with lots of chins. I don't agree with discrimination but if it does happen they've got only themselves to blame. The remedy is in their hands.

I told her that 98 per cent of all weight lost is regained, so how could fat people 'help themselves'?

I don't believe that statistic. Look at the people who go to Weight Watchers. Look at the Slimmers of the Year. When they lose six or eight stones I don't believe they are going to let themselves put it all back on again. That's just a cop-out. If it were true, then doctors would not expect their patients to lose weight if they knew they were going to regain it. It's a question of taking yourself in hand. You won't convince me otherwise.

I have noticed a curious twist to the widespread notion that 'people are fat because they eat too much, or stuff themselves with cream cakes/chocolate'. When thin people eat a great deal, or eat these fat-associated foods, they actually inspire *admiration*. Comments are made: 'Aren't you *marvellous* — you can eat all that and still keep your figure.' They are actually *given credit* as if in some mysterious way they exercise control, not over what they eat, but over their own metabolisms and physiology. It seems to me rather like the principle of it not being the misdemeanour that matters, it's being found out. Any kind, any excess of eating is acceptable as long as the eater does not get fat — or indeed put on any weight at all.

Well, I asked for that, literally, and I reassured Janette that it was good material for the book and that she had not wounded me personally. But of course she had. So many of her very articulate arguments sounded convincing. Everyone seems to know someone who has lost weight and not regained it — or they tell you that they only maintain their own weight by constant discipline. Useless to tell her that most Slimmers of the Year put all that weight back on.

There are some fat women who have an extremely positive and stable body image and I am not intending to leave them out, because those of us who do not share their wholeness in that direction can perhaps learn much from them. But the majority of my large sample of fat women were not happy with their bodies and I feel this needs to be addressed first.

It is difficult to claim autonomy when the odds are so heavily stacked against you. It is extremely difficult to believe 'I am alright. My body is good. There is nothing wrong with my fat. It does not define me as a person' when all around the world is telling us that we have no right to feel like that. The old saying — give a dog a bad name — is relevant here: if you tell someone something often enough and long enough, they will believe it. And this lies at the heart of it all. You must learn to value yourself, say those who wish to help the fat woman repair her damaged psyche. But how? We do not live in emotional isolation, and condemnation and ostracism hit hard. For every tiny step we may take on the path to self-acceptance we are beset by a dozen setbacks of the kind that haunt a fat woman's life, whether it be taunts or practical difficulties yet again drawing attention to our anti-social bodies.

Our self-esteem and therefore our self-image is multi-faceted. We are judged, and so judge ourselves, on the basis of our appearance, our inability to bring ourselves into line with 'normality', our social intrusiveness (taking up more than our share of space) and the problems we cause others (doctors, our husbands, friends, mothers, children).

It is important to understand that the way we perceive ourselves stems directly from the messages we received about ourselves in childhood, including the teenage years. Until we reach maturity, we are dependent on others to give us our self-esteem. What comes from outside starts, in earliest childhood, to build, layer upon layer, our beliefs about ourselves. When we are very young we internalise both approval and disapproval and they become the yardsticks by which we measure ourselves. A fat child will take inside her parents' feelings about her size. This may be in the form of anxiety or disgust — either way the child gets the message that there is something wrong with her. It is reinforced only too easily by school, where no fat child is exempt from the taunts, the jeers, the jibes and the sheer cruelty of her school-fellows. This is often reinforced by teachers who do not value the fat child as highly as the normal, slim active ones. She may begin to get the idea, even at infant school, that she is stupid.

Many women have thin childhoods and start putting on weight around puberty. This is referred to as puppy fat and is devastating when the child has reached the age when it suddenly is important to conform, to start being interested in fashion and hair and boys. Suddenly the other girls are spending a great deal of time in front of the cloakroom mirrors at school and the fat adolescent is caught up in the intense pain of knowing that she is not like them. How great this pain is, and how she copes with being different will depend on the messages she received about herself in childhood. But she hears it now from all sides: 'fat is bad'. She opens newspapers and magazines and finds that famous people who put on weight are viciously attacked. Diets, surgery, all manner of fat-killing treatments proliferate like weeds in women's magazines.

When my daughters were younger they used to have a comic every week with picture serials. There was one about a fat girl who wore glasses (except that in the drawings she was not fat at all, just fatter than the other skinny girls — a dangerous image for impressionable teenage children). Of course, her life was an unhappy mess, derided by schoolteachers and peers alike. But eventually she lost weight (and her glasses disappeared) and how her life changed! All because she became thin. I cancelled the comic.

On August 7th 1989, Anna Kwiatkowski, 32, of Michigan, was shot twice in the head by her father. When arrested, Valentine Kwiatkowski claimed the attempted 'mercy killing' was because of mounting medical bills caused by his daughter's weight (360 lb) and her asthmatic condition. When the two shots did not kill her, her family waited almost two hours before deciding to take her to hospital. Her family portrayed Anna as a disabled woman and a burden, but the hospital where she worked as a volunteer reported her as cheery and happy with no noticeable health problems. On the other hand, neighbours reported that they had seen and heard Anna being physically and verbally abused by her father and sister.

NAAFA Newsletter, September 1989

When I was at school it was the frankly fat girls who were despised. That was in the 1950s and early sixties. Since the sixties' thinness revolution, girls at school are under a new and insidious pressure. It is not enough to be slim — so that a girl of 5'5" weighing nine stones (126 lb) is likely to be called fat. My daughters tell me that everyone describes themselves as fat even when they know they are not. Why? Because thinness is now equated with perfection, and in the eyes of these young women, to claim it would be akin to boasting, so far has our cultural ideal shifted. The increase of anorexia nervosa to epidemic proportions appears not to trouble teenagers or adults. Fear of fatness is a powerful motivator. Anorexia is self-inflicted; unlike the fat woman, the anorexic does not want to give up her body shape. The extremism of the anorexic shape is secretly admired, just as the extreme measures that Victorian women went to, endangering their lives to obtain wasp waists, were admired. '*Il faut souffrir pour être belle*' is being taken far too literally.

> **Starving for Perfection**
> Some of (Dr Dawson's) patients have arrived only a week away from death by self-starvation. All are profoundly disturbed, self-destructive, highly mani-pulative and destructive of their families . . . There is something devilish about these children . . . and they discover that simply by refusing to eat normally, they can drive their parents to despair, they can command attention and control their families' lives. We often glimpse a light of fiendish malice in their eyes, as when Dr Dawson asks 'Why do you want to cause your mother so much pain?' and that smile breaks out, a smile of triumphant power and achievement.
>
> Polly Toynbee's report on anorexic teenage girls, *Radio Times*, 20-26 February 1993

I realize that I am probably making some people very angry by my apparent lack of sympathy for anorexics. I can only reflect my own experiences and those of the other fat women on whose behalf I have researched and written this book. Of course anorexia is an illness. Of course it needs care and attention and treatment. And anorexics get these things. Talking to a large number of people in the medical and psychological professions it becomes clear that there is a deep commitment to the care of anorexics. And an unspoken — in many cases — acknowledgement that they deserve care because they have exercised those admirable qualities, self-control and self-discipline, even though they have become sick through doing so. How often I have heard people say they wouldn't mind a dose of anorexia. However sick, the anorexic has not broken our strict social rules about size and so she invites compassion.

The level of professional interest in anorexia is still growing fast. One specialist in eating disorders told me that it was an area of medicine that people wanted to specialize in because it has aspects of femaleness and childishness that both men and women respond to. The idea of wasting away carries fragile, romanticised undertones and images of Victorian heroines and consumptives taking their last breaths. All these factors combine to bring out the Sir Galahad impulse in both sexes, and they rush forth with all their strength, power and knowledge to rescue these damsels in distress. On the other hand, said my informer, people in the medical profession do not like dealing with obesity because it is unrewarding and because they are so prejudiced.

As Dr Joan Gomez, an expert in eating disorders, says: 'Starving is magic. It's a safe way of rebelling against the pressures, yet no-one can be cross. Controlling your appetite is "good" — but parents are gratifyingly concerned. No one makes demands on a heartbreakingly thin and frail youngster.' Anorexia is not confined to female teenagers, as is often thought. There is 'anorexia tardive' (late onset). Joan Gomez talks of a 50-year-old woman who felt lost. Her mother had died, her children were established in their own lives, her husband was busy with his career. 'Her anorexia made her the focus of attention. Her husband spent hours coaxing her to take a morsel. The children visited her assiduously.'[15]

It is hard for me as a fat woman to feel a great sympathy for the anorexic and that is a difficult thing to handle because I dislike the lack of compassion I find in myself. I would like to mention two incidents which I found distressing, particularly the first one. I was at a local meeting when a woman was brought in in a state of collapse. She sat down at the edge of the room with someone attending to her. I looked at her and realised that she was not going to live for very long. It was the most horrifying and shocking realisation; it really was like looking death in the face. After a while, someone took her arm and led her out. I assumed she had collapsed in the street and guessed that she was in the terminal stages of cancer, but found it strange that no-one sent for a doctor or ambulance.

I was later told that she lived near the house where the meeting was being held and had tried to go for a short walk. She had managed a few yards but had to stop and had come in to sit down. Yes, she was dying, someone told me. She had anorexia, had refused treatment and was now at a stage where her heart or her kidneys were likely to fail any day. She had three small children. She did not usually leave the house now, but very occasionally tried to get some exercise.

My first feeling was immense compassion followed by anger. I still cannot sort one from the other. She had chosen to die, leaving her children. I was assured that no-one could help her. Something in me wanted to go to her, to try to tell her to stop before it was too late. Something very irrational also told me that I, as a fat woman, might have a chance of talking to her, or rather of making her listen. I cannot explain the lack of logic in that. It was related to an identification with extreme suffering, and in a way with death — both death itself and the death of the spirit that can occur when someone is disvalued to such an extent that the whole of life can seem like one long, lonely struggle. That is what it is like for fat people and that is obviously what it has been like for that unknown woman. I still have not resolved my feelings about her — I only know that somehow she and I have a great deal in common.

The second incident concerns one of my closest friends who has lived with a permanent and intractable fear of fatness. She has always been super-thin and has in fact been diagnosed and treated for anorexia. She is sensitive and highly intelligent and aware that it is social pressure that has made her do this to herself. Now cured of anorexia, she still maintains a twig-thin body. She has one daughter and vowed she would not let her daughter suffer as she did. She was going to let her be herself, but she could not help imposing on the girl her obsessive hatred of fatness. The girl became anorexic when she was in her teens and spent months in hospital. My friend is frantic with guilt. She cannot believe that she has done this to her daughter; she cannot explain how she did it. She is a good and loving mother but somehow, in her desire to save her daughter from being the social outcast that she had dreaded becoming herself, though never had, she went over the top.

It is no wonder, that we, the despised fat of the land, sometimes feel we are living in a different world from the one where a small body size is the passport to normal life. Bodysize is a contentious issue, and one that needs tackling head on. Living in a culture that has gone mad has caused slim women to define themselves as fat. A friend of mine, size 12 and just under 6' tall, says she wakes up some mornings and knows that she is going to have to wear a floaty dress because she is too fat for the skirt she might have wanted to wear. She feels she should be a size 10. It isn't empty-headed young girls who say these things; it is mature, intelligent women — like funny, quirky Anne Robinson who presents BBC's *Points of View*, whose own point of view about size and health represents the current obsession in a nutshell: 'I still smoke which is dreadful, but I don't inhale. I wouldn't smoke if I thought that when I stopped I wouldn't put on weight. I desperately battle to be a size 10 and I'm a natural size 12'.[16] Or actress Patricia Hodge, in an interview with Penny Vincenzi:

> She sat down beside me on the sofa, all perfect size 8 of her and said, no, she couldn't possibly have milk in her tea because it was such a ghastly effort these days to keep her weight down. 'I always used to be thin but I have to work hard at it now, it's driving me mad really. I am careful, absolutely careful all the time. I live on salads and fruit and stuff and if I go to a restaurant I never choose the things I really want to eat. And I can't be indifferent to food because I really like it.'[17]

At present I'm 5'7" and freely admit I weigh far too much. I'm vast, dress size 14 . . . I have been known to consume more chocolate and ice-cream than is good for one.

Carol Thatcher, daughter of ex-Prime Minister
Evening Standard, 16 November 1992

When an intelligent and mature woman, who is a 'natural size 12' is prepared to risk her life and health by smoking so that she can continue to 'desperately battle to be a size 10' we can get some idea of why slim women are now constantly defining themselves as 'fat'.

It is a Western sickness, a denial of a woman's body, a desire for a child's body. Indeed, when Justin de Villeneuve discovered Twiggy in the 1960s, it is clear that it was her child's body that captivated him:

> There was this lovely girl, so tiny and so beautiful . . .
> There was this little cockney girl in a little white gown
> with her long neck and her huge, huge eyes — she looked
> like a fawn. She looked like Bambi.[18]

It is far from natural for a woman to be a size 8. But I have
talked to women — intelligent, consciousness-raised,
feminist women — who have admitted to me that what they
really long for is to be a size 6. And I met one who actually
was a size 6 — and she was so *proud* of it. That means a 28″
chest. No breasts. The same size, in fact, as those very
ethereal eleven year olds in the gym on my first day at high
school. A child's size. A *small,* girl-child's size. A far cry
from the other side of the world; in her book *The Politics
of Breastfeeding* Gabrielle Palmer says that women's sexual
attractiveness is not linked with a pre-fertile body shape in
peasant society: 'Indeed in Papua New Guinea there is a
dreaded curse that a witch may put on an enemy to make
her breasts stay pert and upright like a young girl's
forever.'[19]

WHO PERCEIVES WHAT IS FAT?

At the first national conference of the London Fat Women's
Group on 18 March, 1989 there was some controversy over
the presence of a number of women who were quite clearly
not fat. This was a sensitive issue; journalists who had
infiltrated the conference were asked to leave because this
was a coming together of fat women who wished to share
their fears, frustrations and hang-ups just for once without
the presence of thin people. Several women felt extremely
hostile towards these thin women, especially as four
hundred had been turned away due to lack of space. There
was obviously no way the organizers could have checked
the weights of the women who applied to attend; the thin

ones felt they had as much right to be there because *they* defined themselves as fat.

While respecting the painful inner feelings of a woman who is unhappy with her body because *she* judges it to be too fat, there has to be a clear line drawn between self-perception and definition of fatness, and frank overweight. However strong the inner drive towards perfection as perceived in this context, the unhappiness caused by falling below one's *own* standards is not the issue, or at least only part of the issue I am addressing here. This book is about what it means to be fat — fat as recognised by the world, defined as deviant and punished accordingly. When women like Anne Robinson and Patricia Hodge publicly pronounce the essential importance to them of being a size 8 or 10, they are representing a group of women chasing the ideal set for us by anorexic models. That is another matter — it is not the fat woman's problem though that ideal has been the cause for increased stigmatisation as we are moved further and further away from what is set as the cultural norm.

When I started to think about mirrors I realized that I had never had a mirror in my bedroom. This has been the case for so long that I cannot remember when I made a conscious decision not to do so. It is unconscious — when moving house and furnishing my bedroom it has never occurred to me to include a mirror. Then my family complained that there was no mirror in the bathroom; that had not seemed to me to be a grave omission but I took their point and we have a small one above the basin. My daughters both have old-fashioned dressing table mirrors and a full-length mirror was on my youngest daughter's birthday list as she approached seven!

Avoiding mirrors was one of the things agreed on almost unanimously by the women who wrote and spoke to me for the book and it was echoed by the women at the fat women's conference:

When I catch sight of myself unexpectedly in a shop window I feel horror and anger that that monster is really ME.

I feel alright about myself until I look in a mirror. I see someone fat and ugly and have to believe that someone is me. They make me look fatter than I think I am.

I was invited to go and see a friend's new conservatory. It was beautiful and I was looking out at the view when I turned round and realized that the whole of the back wall was one vast mirror. I had caught sight of myself, completely inadvertently, unposed, just as I am — and it was such a grotesque sight I felt upset for hours. I didn't know I was that fat and ugly.

For the same reason, many fat women avoid having their photographs taken. Working for a magazine, I was asked to go to a studio to have a picture taken to accompany my writing. I panicked. When I got there the photographer said: 'We've got hair and make-up here, you can have any look you want for this.' I just said to him: 'Could you light it so that it doesn't show my fat face and all my chins?' The result was a masterpiece of art; the camera may not lie but a good photographer can disguise the truth! I look ten years older, but with what magnificent planes of face, cheeks and chins in shadow. The nicest thing about it was that my family hated it because it was not 'me'. They thought I looked austere and forbidding.

This careful avoidance of confronting ourselves is a nerve-centre for many of us. We, in our bodies, are the monster we are afraid to meet. It is difficult to explain the rationale behind this. We know we are fat, we are told we are ugly, gross, elephantine — we only have to look down at our bodies. Only someone who has known the terror —

and I do not exaggerate — of having to look at themselves will know what I am talking about. I believe it to be a result of early rejection by others. The cruellest taunts of childhood are buried deep in us, probably inaccessible to our conscious minds. We were told in effect that we were deformed monsters, and that took root. That is what our unconscious has absorbed and that is the truth we fear we might find by facing ourselves. While we avoid confrontation, there might still be a chance that it is not as bad as deep down we suspect.

Psychological tests done on fat people's estimation of their own body size have produced different sets of results. One study has shown they persistently overestimate their true limits, another claims they underestimate. It is possible to see how both can be true without contradicting each other. To overestimate is to be possessed by the fear of the monster to a great extent. Literally. To underestimate is to avoid, to hope that it is not true, to feel unable to face the truth. Hilde Bruch talks about fat people as feeling their bodies as external to themselves. They do not identify with this 'bothersome and ugly thing they are condemned to carry through life and in which they feel confined and imprisoned'.[20]

It is true that there is a split between body and spirit. Many fat women find it difficult if not impossible to treat their bodies well. They find it strange to see other women tending to a cut or bruise on their bodies, for example. The fat woman is more likely to feel any wound is 'deserved'. As for the women's magazines that suggest you 'Pamper your body', it would seem almost sinful. What is there in this body that makes it deserving of care? They perceive it as the outward and visible sign of their inner and sinful nature that created it. Again, it goes back to received, repeated conditioning: fat is self-inflicted. The remedy is in your own hands. If you remain fat it continues to be proof that you do not have the basic qualities of decency that entitle you to be a fully paid-up member of the human race as we see it in our culture.

So a fat woman is unlikely to notice her clear skin, or her well-shaped hands. She will see the little hill of flesh nudging her watchstrap, the way her thighs spread across the whole chair when she sits down. This body is not for loving. It is for punishing. I confess that I have on many occasions bumped into a sharp corner and bruised myself quite hard (the edge of a desk perhaps). Almost unconsciously, as the pain and the bruising appear, a voice within says: 'Good. You deserve that.'

I do not believe that we do this to ourselves. We perpetuate the messages we are given in our formative years. We internalise them and repeat them back to ourselves even while they are still being hurled at us. This came from a desperately distressed middle-aged woman:

> I'm fat, gross, overweight, obese. I cannot accept my size. I have no wise and witty retort for those who comment on my appearance. Instead I burn up, then weep. How can I accept such ugliness?

How can we change our own self-image and 'meet the monster'? It is a frequent metaphor in mythology that the monster we run from is the one to fear. The one we turn and face often changes into something lovely.

Our uneasiness with our bodies is summed up in the pithy little epigrams most people are so familiar with:

> Imprisoned in every fat man a thin one is wildly signalling to be let out. (Cyril Connolly).

> I'm fat, but I'm thin inside. Has it ever struck you that there's a thin man inside every fat man, just as they say there's a statue inside every block of stone? (George Orwell).

and the converse of that — the thing we live in fear of as encapsulated by Kingsley Amis: 'Inside every fat man there's an even fatter one trying to get out.'

These small pieces of 'wisdom' have become incorporated into the sayings of our common language.

These quotable quotes are all by men and it is interesting to see the way in which they have removed themselves, the 'I', by referring to the thin man, or the fatter man in the third person, thus distancing themselves from what they have said and leaving a witty but impersonal impression. Is this the essence of the different ways that women and men regard their fatness?

The late Hattie Jacques, known and loved for her comedy roles in film and television portraying matronly characters, always gave off an air of confidence. But she was shy and sensitive about her size and once said: 'When you're my size you're conditioned from childhood to people making jokes against you. You have to make them laugh with you, not at you.'[21] Her words represent the fat woman's dichotomy. We cannot and should not continue in this state of stress, trying to free the 'thin man' and fighting to keep the 'even fatter one' at bay. We have to find a way to love ourselves for the sake of our health and our integrity.

But most of us just try again and again to remove the hated fat.

4

Friends, lovers and mothers

The American chat show *Donahue,* an audience
participation, transatlantic version of BBC's *Kilroy,*
addressed the issues of weight, image and sex in a show
transmitted in the UK in a late night slot. It was soul-baring
time. Responses were mixed, from 'It's great' — from a very
large, vivacious woman — to considerably more shrinking
revelations. So what about the men? asked our no-holds-
barred-let's-get-to-the-root-of-this-one, host. Did they
like sex with large, *cuddly* women? Some sheepishly
admitted that they did. It was all a bit coy until a woman
told of her husband and his friends who used to go out and
find large women and do them the favour of having sex
with them. This was pure altruism, we were led to
understand, because otherwise these unfortunate women
would probably have remained virgins. No pleasure in this
for the men, of course. In fact they referred to such acts as
'mercy missions'. Even the garrulous Donahue was
momentarily lost for words.

We are never so vulnerable as when we are naked — it is
then that fear of the judgement of others and the need for
approval are silently clamorous. When we take off our
clothes for sex we are implying a trust in the way the other
person will treat our bodies, will react to the sight of our
imperfections and will cherish what we are offering of our
most intimate selves. It is perfectly possible to imagine with

reasonable accuracy how a size 12 body looks when naked — we are, after all, frequently treated to the sight of 'perfect' breasts and gently curving hips in films and television sex. But the fat woman's body is her own secret. While clothes can provide an optical illusion, or an elaborate series of them — strong uplift bras, constricting corsets (yes, women do still wear them) and flowing dresses which hide some of the bulges — the stripping of these disguises reveals a body that does not conform in any way with the modern sexual stereotype we have been media-fed.

A mildly overweight woman will be embarrassed by the padding on her hips, the fullness of her breasts, her spare tyre and the bulges of upper arms and inner thighs. For the very fat woman her naked body is a nightmare fantasy which she tries to avoid seeing as much as possible. Huge pendulous breasts with nipples pointing directly to the floor, vast cushions of hips and several tyres. Many fat women cannot even see their own pubic hair because of what is known medically as the 'apron' — the sagging stomach which hangs down, sometimes to the thighs, hence its name. And while most women are sensitive about the sight of scars on their body, the fat woman is criss-crossed with them in every direction, on every part — the stretch marks, silver for the old ones, livid reddish-purple when new weight is gained. Small wonder, then, that sex for the larger woman is one of the most painful areas of her life and one which provoked many tears in the women who talked to me about it:

I try to avoid undressing in front of a partner and don't like 'doing it' with the light on. The men I fancy almost always reject me because they can't overcome their revulsion, despite 'loving me as a person'.

I put on weight after the children were born and when I got to seventeen stones my husband just said he could not bear to have sex with me any more. We haven't made love for two years, I haven't been able to lose weight and our marriage is breaking up. He says he cannot bear to touch me sexually. I think my weight has greatly affected relationships and that it makes me less desirable than when I was slim. My first two marriages failed because of my size and my third marriage is very loving, but not very sexual, due to my size.

The concept of being sexually undesirable because of their weight figured strongly in the majority of the detailed interviews I conducted with large women. Apart from agonising experiences of rejection, I discovered a lowering of expectations. Women felt they were risking too much rejection by even contemplating a relationship with the sort of man they wanted:

I was working in a supermarket and the manager took me home one night. We stopped by a field and lay down together and he screwed me — I'm sorry, but there's just no other way to put it. There was no foreplay, no consideration of my feelings or needs — but I thought that was the nearest to 'love' I would get. We did it twice more after that.

My relationships with men were unsatisfactory as I constantly accepted 'second best' because I did not feel confident enough to get involved with men I was attracted to for fear of rejection because I was too fat.

I feel my size only entitled me to relationships with 'second-class people' — I would not aspire to someone I really wanted because I would assume that *they* could not bear me.

This is a circular situation which can only be broken by women acquiring self-esteem and confidence in their sexuality. While they are prepared to accept second best — whatever that may mean for them — those arrogant men who talked about going on 'mercy missions' will continue to claim their place in sexual politics. If women cannot believe they deserve more, then sex for them will be like 'squirting jam into a doughnut', as Germaine Greer so graphically put it and as Susan's boss, the supermarket manager, demonstrated.[1]

But how to break the circle is one of the most difficult issues that fat women have to tackle. We are fed up with being told to love ourselves when we receive messages of hate from all around. It is the standard psychologist's remark: 'You must learn to love yourself before you can expect anyone to love you.' Yet none of these experts seems able to tell us *how* to love and value ourselves when the world is telling us we've gone wrong, we're a bad lot.

To try to illustrate how agonising and difficult it is for fat women to love themselves and acquire self-esteem, I would like to look at a slim woman's feelings about fatness. Gail is thin, tall, elegant and rather beautiful in a dreamy, almost other-worldly sort of way. She has been my friend for about twenty years and has been one of the very few who has never encouraged me to diet; the reverse in fact, for whenever I have said I was going to lose weight, she has always countered with a protest, because she loves the bodies of large women and thinks I am right as I am. She thinks I would be devaluing myself by changing my body in response to social pressure. Gail is one of the people who make me feel good about myself, because of the sincerity of what she says and because she cares about me as a whole, with my fatness, not in spite of it. She is also one of the most non-judgemental people I know. Yet I sensed that in spite of her very real endorsement of my body, and her occasionally expressed slight envy of what she calls my 'presence', that she herself had a horror of being fat. I asked her about it.

I have a desperate need to fit into one of the media stereotypes. I wouldn't mind not being so thin as long as I still fitted something acceptable; for instance I would not mind having big breasts and curvaceous hips because that would mean I was a voluptuous woman — still an acceptable stereotype.

I am very appearance conscious. I'm always worrying about what I look like. When I look in the mirror I see horrible fat, flabby thighs. I've *always* watched my weight. Once I got hepatitis and I was really thin, like a skeleton and I knew I was too thin. But I got enormous pleasure out of wearing a belt over a jumper because my waist was *so* small. Then when I was better I started putting weight back on. I went to the doctor one day and he said, 'You've put on weight' — meaning that I was better from the illness; he was congratulating me in a way. I had only gone back to the size I was before, but I heard his remark as a condemnation and I was so humiliated. I couldn't face him again after that so I actually changed doctors.

I think it must stem from the fact that I had 'puppy fat' as a child. I remember being at school, aged about twelve, and being unhappy, and of course the other children went on about me being fat. I found it torture, real persecution and I internalised it all and I suppose it's all still there though of course I know that I'm not fat.

It does affect relationships. I remember once going away for a weekend with a lover. He said to me: 'I really like skinny women,' and I was mortified because I thought he meant I wasn't thin enough, that I was failing him by being fat. It ruined the weekend. Now, looking back, I can see that what he was saying, of course, was that he liked *me* because I *was* thin.

Gail is sensitive but not neurotic and has never suffered from bulimia or anorexia. She is psychologically stable. She recognizes that her bad feelings about her body stem from the persecution she suffered in adolescence. She also knows the difference between these internalised feelings which make some situations painful for her, and the persecution that fat women suffer and which she has never had to endure.

I wanted to write about Gail because her feelings show how insecure women can feel about their bodies and about relationships even though they do not cross the boundary into being 'unacceptable'. How much more difficult it is for women who not only bear the internal feelings of shame, hatred and ugliness but also have those feelings affirmed from outside. The combination is so potent that it is very common for a fat woman to view with total mistrust someone who falls in love with her, finds her attractive, wants a relationship, wants to sleep with her, wants to make love to her fat body. It reminds me irresistibly of Groucho Marx saying he wouldn't want to join any club that would accept *him* as a member; it is that exactly.

I really despise people who say they fancy me. I mean, what's wrong with them that they can't do any better for themselves?

I just don't believe it if someone fancies me. I think they're sending me up and I react with total suspicion, sometimes hostility.

Starting a relationship is awful, you keep asking and asking for reassurance that they really do fancy you like this, and of course it's the need for reassurance that can screw the relationship up. But you don't realize that, so you think you've failed again because of the fat.

If someone likes me enough to want a relationship with me, I lose my respect for them. I suppose I can't respect myself, so I transfer that feeling to anyone who seems to feel good things about me. And then I feel angry, I think 'You can't do any better for yourself so you'll content yourself with me'. And I've told people to push off, because I'd rather have nobody than be someone's second or third, fourth, fifth best.

I've never managed a good relationship yet. When a bloke says he likes my body, I scream at him, I call him a liar. Look, I've been called names for years, I've been called a fat cow and a fat bitch, so why should someone come along who doesn't think that? But for all I know, I may have lost someone who really did like me as I am. How do you get round years of abuse and negative conditioning?

I've had two really good relationships — I'm in one of them now. But it never feels secure. The way I've done it is to give them hell — deliberately. If they stick with me through that I know they must really want me. But I hate myself for doing it. It's almost as though if I don't I'll never know the truth about the relationship. I am surprised anyone has stayed with me though, I've been really nasty, just to get them to prove themselves. I think they must have understood why I was doing it — I did try to explain.

There is no easy answer to these deeply ingrained feelings which have usually been there for a long time. Some women are lucky; they find an acceptance of their bodies within a relationship where they are truly loved, though it takes a considerable time for this to happen. It can be the start of a healing process though, the warmth that floods through you bringing you back to life and out of the clutches of the Snow Queen as represented by the cold censure of social prejudice; self-love and acceptance can begin this way.

As with most aspects of weight prejudice, the woman who fears sexual rejection has some grounds for doing so. It is not enough simply to state that if you feel good about yourself you project that feeling and consequently that in itself brings about acceptance. While good self-esteem can to some extent affect the way others regard us, it is a fact that a fat body can be a sexual turn-off as clearly demonstrated by the stated preferences of those who want a slim figure in their sexual partner. The whole subject of sex, sensuality and enjoyment is confused by aesthetics, convention and fear of being different. Those factors influence choice perhaps more than anything else. Many men, especially young men, do not want to be seen with a fat woman. It looks, to their peer groups, as though that were the best they could do for themselves — it hardly needs to be said that a man seen with a tall, slim, shapely blonde is going to command respect and envy and boost his image in their eyes.

Ex-racing driver Niki Lauda who set up his own airline, Lauda Air said:

> I have the most beautiful air hostesses in the world on my planes — I hand pick them all myself. But if they put on weight they are grounded to slim. Either that or they have to be fired. I don't want fat women ruining my reputation.[2]

Strangely enough the above news item does not make me see red. A man who needs that amount of validation must have a very damaged identity.

High performance is increasingly important to men. In this era of high achievement they need expressed recognition of their success and along with cars, expense accounts, gold American Express cards they feel they need the working equivalent of the 'sexy girl on the bonnet' featured at motor shows and in car advertisements. As men climb high in their chosen profession, their wives become more and more of a status symbol — a possession to be flaunted along with their material gains. Just as an executive would die rather than be seen arriving at the office in a beaten up Citroen 2CV, so he would equally refute the idea of having to present a fat wife at cocktail parties and other business/social functions. This is a serious matter to men on the success ladder, as can be seen if you look at the way companies have different gradings of cars according to seniority. His competence and position are assessed by his assets, and such competence would be called into question if he could not obtain or maintain a slim wife. In the business world a wife cannot expect to be given any higher value than any of the other symbols, considerably less when you think of the way some men regard their cars.

As a fat child growing up in a sparsely populated country district I found myself the only one in my neighbourhood facing the problems of being overweight. I became socially isolated around the age of fifteen when the others started having boyfriends. My mother, who was fiercely protective, did not help me to face the harsh facts — that 'nobody loves a fat girl'. She insisted that I had a good figure and that everyone else was too thin. She also told me that personality mattered more than looks and of course she was right — but she omitted to tell me what I was already seeing all around me, that looks, in the shape of 'normal' size, were the first prerequisite for a teenage love-life. It was then that I learnt the powerlessness of being fat. I knew I was not facially unattractive, yet all around me thin girls, whom I could see to be much plainer than I was, were apparently having no difficulty in 'going out' with someone.

I was desperate to conform and at one point played the 'second-best' game — the only boy who showed an interest was considerably educationally sub-normal and rather weird, so there was little conversation, but he was someone to talk about, to be going out with. A lot of the boys enjoyed talking to me like a sister and I latched on to the fact that at least I was wanted in *some* way — and so grew up with a reputation for being a good listener, a comforter. It is something I have to this day and I still do not know if it is really 'me' or an acquired part of the compensating personality fat people build up.

I was lucky in the end — I met my husband when I was nineteen (and, in fact, not too fat) and we have spent twenty-six happy years together. I was slim (for me) on my wedding day — it would have seemed to me, at that time in my life, profane to have been fat — and of course I was much admired for the results of a year's rigorous dieting. The first ten years of my marriage were enclosed by the (chosen) boundaries of home and motherhood, but then I went back to work, several stones heavier. I worked for the BBC which seemed at first a frightening, dangerous world, where on the surface programmes were made, while underneath currents of sexual rivalry, competition and innuendo hummed like air waves. I learnt at once that I was not considered part of this conspiracy, though I got on well with most of my colleagues of both sexes. My best friend, a lovely and talented woman, was quite open in the flaunting of her legs — by means of short, slit skirts — and her breasts — by going bra-less and wearing low-cut see-through blouses. The director's couch legend is no less true for being a legend, and while my friend did no more than sit on the knees of producers she wanted to work with, there were many others who did far more. I suppose in a way it was easier for me not having that pressure, but it meant I had to work a lot harder to get my work noticed.

It was while I was at the BBC that I discovered the hypocritical double standard of men's desires. I was not flirted with or propositioned, did not have to fend off the men while on location. But — *in vino veritas est*, and at the famous drunken BBC Christmas parties I discovered that these men, who did not want to be *seen* with me, certainly lost no opportunity for an attempted grope, making it quite clear what they wanted. I laugh at the irony that I could have gone to bed with a number of men who would not have considered me at all good for their image when sober. I laugh — but for many women the discovery of that truth is a painful one and one that highlights the whole ugly business of men objectifying women.

There is though, I think, another side to this double standard that is worth considering — and that is sex itself, what it is and what it means. In the privacy of the bedroom, image cannot exist, but the motives for choosing a sexual partner are many and complex, and often largely unconscious. And while going around with someone places a self-conscious emphasis on looks, making love is to do with touch and feelings. A great many men have admitted to me that they do like a woman to be 'cuddly' in bed, that they like something to get their arms round and to be enfolded by . . . They like to cup a full breast in their hand rather than to stroke the flat 'poached eggs' that are the breasts of thin women lying down . And somewhere in their deep unconscious lies the memory of a time when breasts and arms and belly were much larger than they were, and that largeness came with warmth and food and satiety. So for many men (and women) the act of sex with a large woman contains the return to mother, symbolically, hidden memories and perhaps longings for their own mother, and primitive yearnings towards the universal Earth Mother. In her we can be lost, enveloped, swallowed. There is a merging of flesh that is difficult to achieve with a thin person, and especially with two thin people where the boundaries of their bodies remain more clearly defined and therefore separate and where pelvic bones can dig in sharply and painfully, where a tight embrace meets not yielding flesh but hard bone, pointed shoulder blades and frangible ribs.

In his book *Till We Have Faces,* which is a recreation of the myth of Cupid and Psyche, C.S. Lewis muses on the nature of love and postulates that to be loved is to be devoured, that maybe loving and devouring are the same thing.[3] In the story Psyche is left in the wilderness, chained to a tree, to be devoured by wild beasts or to be rescued by a lover. That element is literal but the symbolism arising from it touches deep fears and longings. It may be that the feeling of being devoured, swallowed in the body of a large woman, is why some men love sex with her and why some fear it, though they do not recognise it as fear. It then manifests as repugnance, but the repugnance itself begs several questions. Why should someone actually prefer hardness to softness, bones to flesh, if not on account of fear?

Apart from that there is the incest taboo which lurks deep in all of us. If we accept that a large, full, soft body may remind us unconsciously of our mothers, then the sex act may well be repugnant for that reason. For those men who are unable to make love to their wives when they grow fat, help is needed, expert, sensitive, professional help — for them, not their wives. It is they who have the problem.

I was once very surprised to be told by a chauvinist, stereotypical and apparently cold-blooded Anglican vicar that he found women terrifying. Why? Because we literally carry the power to choose to continue or to end the human race. This man feared feminism and any hint of women's solidarity. Just suppose, his thinking ran, that there was a revolution and women decided to take the whole matter of fertility and reproduction entirely into their own hands. Men are absolutely helpless. That was why he appeared to dislike women so much. He really was greatly afraid of our power. He could identify more readily with thin, androgynous women with childlike bodies; the absence of the blatant shape of fertility was reassuring to him. But large women with their hips and stomachs, their big breasts, always reminded him of his primitive fear and he could never be comfortable with them. His wife was a story-book, submissive vicar's wife, her body that of a disciplined ballerina.

I like the metaphor for women's power as demonstrated in the James Bond film *The Living Daylights* where a man is literally crushed to death between a huge woman's breasts. The part was played by Julie T. Wallace who also played the deserted wife in Fay Weldon's television adaptation of her novel *Life and Loves of a She-Devil.*[4] Julie was required to put on three stones for her part in the series — to emphasize her power. When her husband cheated on her, the 'woman scorned' was magnificent in her size and strength and her husband, played by Dennis Waterman, impotent in his weedy smallness. It was of course a parody, but it leaves us with questions about men's feelings about the power of women.

So men always seem ambivalent in their desires. One type for their image, one for their bed.

WHAT *DO* MEN FEEL ABOUT BIG WOMEN?

I heard you were writing a book about fat women and wondered if you could give me any advice. I work for a company making floor tiles and have often had to deal with a man from another firm on the telephone. We have always got on well, but recently there has been an extra something in our conversations — first, they became more personal as we told each other about our lives, now there is an unmistakable intimacy. We are very attracted to each other, if you can understand that. He keeps saying what a lovely personality I've got, and how you can really get to know someone over the phone because you are listening to the overtones in their voice and not being distracted by their appearance or mannerisms. Now he wants us to meet, and he has made it obvious that he thinks we are already half-way to a relationship. The thing is, I feel the same, but I am terrified of meeting him because I am fat. We have touched briefly on appearances, just to get a mental picture of each other but I was too much of a coward to tell him the truth. We have been getting to know each other on the phone for about a year now and it feels really comfortable. I do feel that we would enjoy each other and maybe it could turn serious. I do get more than ordinary pleasure out of talking to him — there's definitely something else. Do I risk telling him I'm fat and turn him off me? Or do I arrange the meeting and just turn up? If I tell him first, he may not even want to give it a try. But if I don't — and he hates fat women I don't think I could cope with the rejection. Should I just leave things as they are — a telephone friendship? But if I do, I risk missing something deeper.

There is no kind of reassurance that I or anyone else can give this woman that her fears are groundless. Even though this man has already got to know her personality and is attracted to it, fat hatred and fear are so very powerful that the knowledge of her size *may* affect his evaluation of her. Many people would not blame him, though if he does find her fatness unacceptable he will be aware that he is the loser. But he, as much as she, is a victim of cultural pressure and I cannot really advise this unhappy woman, other than to tell her to risk it because we attain nothing if we are afraid of risk.

A close friend of mine has a very happy marriage and no problems with sex. She and her husband are able to joke about it; both virgins when they married, he says he has never known anything else and is very happy with love-making. He admits to enjoying the voluptuousness of holding a full and fleshy body and says he would hate to feel bones. Outside the bedroom things are very different. He is the managing director of a firm with the high-pressure social life that sort of job requires. She is the managing director's wife and required to be an adjunct to him at dinner parties and other such social/business functions. She always felt uncomfortable at these and assumed it was because she was fat and the other women there were despising her. While there was almost certainly truth in her idea that she was being negatively evaluated, it took several years before she realised that her feeling of being unacceptable was stemming from her husband's discomfort at having a fat wife, though he was barely aware of it himself. She challenged him with this notion and for a long time he denied it. After many painful hours of trying to work through this, during which their marriage became decidedly shaky, he was able to face his own prejudice which he had buried, as he loved his wife and did not want to admit the thing that deep down he knew was there. Then he finally confessed, ashamed and unhappy, that he would prefer her to be slim. Just as so many women cannot find the autonomous self-confidence to fly in the face of social pressure, so some men cannot handle the assumed insult to their maleness by being seen with one of the 'second-class citizens'. And while I cannot endorse the Niki Lauda philosophy of life, that he does not want 'fat women ruining my reputation', there is a vast gap between that and my friend's husband, caught in a cultural maelstrom.

This couple solved the immediate problem with a joky compromise, though I suspect it cannot be a real solution. My friend simply refused to attend any more social events as the managing director's wife. If he felt ashamed of her, she said, she would remove the cause of his shame. He attends them alone or takes his sister where there is a specific requirement for a female. This means that he has to take the responsibility for explaining the permanent absence of his wife. She is freed from the misery of attending events where she felt threatened and says she is quite happy with the arrangement. But unless the root of all this is tackled, I cannot see how their marriage can survive without being eroded in some way. Again, the problem is his, not hers. He needs to learn, through therapy, self-awareness, building on his own self-esteem, that his worth as a man does not depend on his wife's weight.

Marje Proops, in her agony column in the *Daily Mirror*, gives the 'go-ahead' to a husband about to commit adultery on the grounds that his wife is obese. She adds: 'But don't forget that poor disabled creature at home, clearly unable to control her need to gorge — as much a cripple as anyone you'll see in a wheelchair.' Offending obese women and the disabled in one fell swoop — call that 'advice'? Sounds more like agony to us.

Cosmopolitan's 'Misogynist of the Month', March 1992

Society would have it the other way round, though, and always has done. We have always been taught that we have a duty to look our best for our men; that is part of the objectifying of women that has been going on for centuries. There have always been double standards about men's and women's appearances. Women are expected to shave underarm and leg hair, men are not, for example. And it is comparatively recently that deodorants for men have been introduced; there are still a lot of the brutes who would not dream of applying anything so apparently effeminate. The hunky, macho image includes a beefy body, but women are supposed to 'keep their figure' for their man. This sickening propaganda comes mainly from women's magazines, so it is hardly surprising when men write to Problem Pages with letters like the following:

> My wife knows I prefer her slim and she struggled with her weight until a few months ago when she announced she would no longer diet and I had to accept her as she was. She is happier and easier to live with but I do find it difficult to accept that she will never be slim again.

Could anything be more crass and self-centred? And it is fat people that are said to be self-indulgent!

Even when a relationship is apparently good, it seems that it is rarely truly unconditional:

> I'm in a stable, serious relationship — in fact we live together. I feel undesirable and hate to undress in front of my boyfriend. My size has not yet affected this relationship. My boyfriend is very understanding and says I should learn to love myself, but he would rather I was slim.

This rather sad letter made me very angry. The woman is responding to the usual feelings of pressure about her size in her feelings of undesirability. I find her use of the word 'yet' extremely poignant — it tells whole stories in itself. No wonder she uses it, though, when in an apparently secure relationship where her boyfriend is 'very understanding' and thinks she should learn to love herself, he would also prefer her to be slim. And how dare he be understanding when fat women need the men who profess to love us to celebrate us, the whole of us, our fat bodies, not to patronise us by 'understanding'.

> I'm still looking for a man who will excite me as much as a baked potato.
>
> From Henry Jaglom's film *Eating*

There is an idea abroad that husbands should be there with the whip, keeping our dieting and bodycare up to the mark. Having our best interests at heart, it's called. If they don't do this, the theory runs, they are undermining our endeavours; even, as one magazine suggested, bent on sabotage. Watch out for this, the warning goes, and don't be a pawn in his game. Where one couple had separated, the magazine suggested that the husband was not the criminal but the accessory after the fact, the facts being that his wife had cared too little about herself and eaten too much. The writer goes on to say that her own partner has been known to 'shoot her down in flames' (what a violent metaphor) — telling her she needed to diet when all she wanted to be told was that she looked like a million dollars (with of course, the implicit inference that she could not look that good *unless* she dieted).

But, the writer goes on to say gratefully, there is a big plus to this approach: he is the first to encourage me when I do manage to shed a few pounds. And I'm grateful, honestly (who is she trying to convince with her use of the word 'honestly?' Methinks . . .), that not only does he want for me what I want for myself, but that he is not prepared to lie to me, though I could wish now and then that he were not so brutally frank. Oh, yes, thank goodness he doesn't want me to be fat. Why would any man want his wife or girlfriend to be fat? Husbands, the writer goes on to say, are in essence a danger to us. They may not keep us up to the mark. 'The very aspects of marriage which we most value, the cosiness, the closeness, the *acceptance* (my italics) can militate against a sustained campaign of self-improvement.'

There is nothing like a new, slender you to rekindle the romance in your relationship says the dieters' folk wisdom. Val, who lost three stones and felt that her marriage had been 'revitalised' admits: 'There's a tendency to think, "If you don't love me first thing in the morning with no make-up and stale breath and with my hair all over the place, then you don't love me at all".' Quite. Val goes on: 'I used to be quite bloody minded about it . . . and my attitude would be: "Well it's the essential me, the person that's important, not how I look at this moment".' Good for you Val, now you're talking about *real* feelings. But she wasn't of course. After that last statement when it looked as though she was reaching out for integrity, Val realises the error of her ways: 'It's a pretty stupid attitude . . . If I like myself far more now I'm size 12, why shouldn't Keith feel the same?' I despair when I read things like this because they are written in publications by women and for women and they collude absolutely with the social sickness which is now all pervasive. It is one thing to accept the truth that we as fat women have a hard time of it out there in the world; there is some kind of rationale for encouraging us to slim in order to escape the pain of stigma and prejudice. But I find something sick in the promotion of the idea that in personal intimate relationships our worth, our qualification for love, in fact, is dependent on our body size and shape.[5]

American researchers Stuart and Jacobson have come to the conclusion that many husbands actually *want* their wives to be fat, but don't get hopeful — this has nothing to do with loving soft flesh and generous curves. According to this pair it suits men to keep their spouses oppressed and plump, to camouflage their own seedy, socially deviant activities. Like being out on the town, drinking, sleeping around, while their wives, fat and impotent, remain stuck miserably in the home. And of course men do not feel threatened, apparently, by a fat wife; no chance of her taking a lover. Their research also shows that marriage itself makes you fat — an average weight gain of 18.4lbs in thirteen years for happily married women, and as much as 42.6lbs in an unhappy marriage. The reason, they claim, is that women who have 'passed the test' of having to prove themselves attractive and sexually desirable (they have after all, caught their man and proved they are lovable) then relax and, heaven forbid, let go of their weight control. Husbands, while appearing to support their wives' efforts to lose weight, deliberately sabotage them by 'bringing home ice-cream and candy and telling me I had to stop dieting'. In this way, they keep their wives imprisoned, claim the authors, rather like the wicked witch in Hansel and Gretel.[6]

This is a complex theory which would appear to carry some truth. In the famous fattening houses for brides in Africa, for example, it is the greatest privilege to be a chosen bride, consigned to two years or so of being fed the most awful, fattening foods and finally emerging very fat indeed. This is often interpreted as preparing the most beautiful of brides in a culture that values fatness but it does have sinister undertones. There is an ulterior motive — to render these women powerless. And we know that in Western Society when women get fat many of them cease to feel sexually attractive. But this does not apply in a culture where fatness is valued.

My husband cannot get an erection and after a lot of heartache he confessed it was because he was repulsed by my size — I have put on three stones in five years.

I discovered that my husband had been having an affair with another woman. When I challenged him about it, he said that he loved me but he longed for a slim, sexy body for love-making. He said he never intended to get into an affair, but was finding sex with me a turn-off.

The man I had been living with for ten years finally left me. He was sorry, he said, but he just had not been able to come to terms with my fat body, despite 'loving me as a person'.

My boyfriend left me after a two year relationship which had not been very sexually satisfactory. When he finally decided to go he was very bitter, and said that because of my refusal to lose weight I had ruined both our lives.

So maybe there is some currency in Stuart and Jacobson's contentions that men have their reasons for keeping their women fat. Either to do what they like to 'compensate' for an unattractive partner or as an excuse to end a relationship without taking any responsibility.

There is another possibility, though maybe I am being fanciful. A *Weight Watchers* article called 'Check your mate'[7] makes many of the same sort of suggestions about husbands sabotaging their wives' diets. Both Stuart and Jacobson's book and the article are saying clearly, 'Watch out. *He* could have his reasons for wanting you to be fat'. And Richard Stuart, co-author of the research on husbands and weight, is a 'psychological director' of Weight Watchers International.[8] In their book, after revealing their findings, Stuart and Jacobson devote much of their writing to the business of — you've guessed it — losing weight.

For me, the similarity between the book and the Weight Watchers magazine message invalidates much of the evidence. Obviously in both there is a vested interest in losing weight and therefore in Weight Watchers. There is no mention of the men who truly like their women to be fat. Those who would have us slim would refute the idea that there are such men in our culture. But there are, usually men in a lower socio-economic class who do not place the same value on achievement and possessions as their class-conscious, ambitious and socially mobile brothers. Or they are men working in non-competitive professions who do not need a woman as part of their image package. Or the 'new men' often derided as being wimpish — those who feel strong concern for the future of mankind and planet earth, who subscribe to green politics, whose priorities lie in issues like pacifism, concern about the Third World, pollution.

I will be accused of generalising — and I can think of at least one green politician who abhors fat women! But it is impossible to make these points without generalising to a certain degree and it would appear that those whose philosophy of life embraces acceptance of people's inner beauty, however idealistic that may seem, are those who look beyond the shallow dictates of society, and who very often are in the process of rebelling against it. The establishment as we know it today under the government we have, with its emphasis on acquisition and achievement and its lack of compassion and humanitarian ideals, is the same society that says no to fat women and yes to life-threatening technology in the name of progress:

> I fought in the sixties against racism. I campaigned for employers to include gays and disabled people. I would be a rotten sort of hypocrite if I rejected fat women. My wife was slim when we got married, but has put on weight over twelve years and is now fat by any definition. How can that make any difference to the way I feel about her? She has blossomed with maturity into a lovely,

compassionate woman, sensitive to the needs and hurts of others. We are very conscious of how lucky we are with our marriage.

I didn't marry my wife for her body or her money — if our relationship had been dependent on either, I wouldn't have married her at all! Isn't it the person inside that counts?

OK, sometimes when we're out I feel a bit embarrassed when people stare because my wife is large. Then I think, what have I got to be so smug about? I'm not exactly perfect.

My girlfriend is fat and she really hates it. But I see how much hurt she suffers from being rejected and laughed at, and it just makes me want to protect her and make sure she knows there is one place where she is perfect as she is — with me. I mean, she wouldn't be a different person if she were slim.

I'm proud of what being fat has done to my wife. Because she has experienced so much persecution, she is very aware of the pain of anyone who doesn't fit. I don't know if she would have had that degree of compassion otherwise. The one certain thing is that she could never make unkind remarks about anyone else, and that sets her apart in my opinion.

My wife has put on a lot of weight — gone from eight to seventeen stone in ten years. She is marvellously attractive, does not want to diet and would not be seen dead in any of these clothes that are meant to be flattering, whatever that means. Wearing a bikini in Italy last summer, she had no shortage of admirers. I find nothing so tedious as a load of women yakking on about their latest diets.

Or, as author Anthony Burgess told presenter Sue Lawley on the *Wogan* show in March 1989, 'I once went to bed with a top model. It was like going to bed with a bicycle'.

I suspect that the truth about what men really want in a woman's body and what they think they ought to *say* they want will remain shrouded in their own self-consciousness until men stop seeing women as objects or accessories.

In a survey conducted by *Singles* magazine[9] to find out the top ten attributes that men look for in women, being slim came third in order of priority. It was ranked higher than being a non-smoker, or intelligent, loving, affectionate, caring and humorous. So are we to deduce that men want a cold, unloving, undemonstrative, uncaring, dim-witted, humourless smoker — as long as she is slim? The survey did not analyse whether the importance of these qualities was for the purpose of a woman as a partner in a relationship or just a superficial appraisal — the features a man would like to be visible as he parades her in public as a symbol and a possession. There is ambivalence and paradox contained in this but I would see little hope for the future of humanity if slimness really was carefully considered and rated to be more important in a relationship than those other qualities.

An American study found that college students placed a fat person very low on the list of desirable partners, stating that they would prefer to marry an embezzler, cocaine user, ex-mental patient, shop-lifter, sexually promiscuous person, communist, drug user or atheist.[10] I suppose the factor to take into account here is that these were college students, and I know from my own children that young people of that age are fiercely image-conscious and competitive, and though they might be quite happy to have fat people as friends, their own sense of identity and self-worth is still too unformed and fragile to dare to depart from peer-group norms.

There is a dating agency in the UK called 'Plump Partners' founded in 1986 by Sandy Millington. Sandy sets no limits on requirements for her prospective clients and has discovered that while 90 per cent of the women who approach her are bruised and damaged by previous rejections, two thirds of the men on her books are slim. They have joined her agency because they choose to look for a large woman and Sandy has seen several successful matches between fat women and thin men, without any of the demeaning overtones so often suggested in low-brow television comedy. One man once travelled two hundred miles to meet Sandy herself and although they got on very well, she was too thin for him at thirteen stone — one of the few occasions, Sandy says, that she regrets no longer weighing the nineteen stone she once did, though she is now engaged to one of her clients — a slim man. Both of them are *very* happy.

Sandy started the agency after a painful divorce. She joined dating agencies and her phone started ringing. But the talk always got round to her appearance. She laid her thirteen stones on the line and found that the phone was put down as quickly as minimal courtesy allowed. She met a fat girl who turned up for a blind date in a pub. The man she was meeting turned up, said 'I can't be seen with you,' threw a five pound note down on the table and walked out. Sandy was terrified of something like that happening to her — then she read about a dating agency for fat people in America, and being a resourceful person she started her own.

Now Plump Partners has more than fourteen hundred people on its books, a monthly bulletin for members and weights are recorded so that no one need fear rejection on that score. Running Plump Partners has given Sandy a wealth of insight into the pain experienced by women wanting a relationship but afraid of rejection on account of their size. Most of these have gone through those painful experiences and need a great deal of counselling in order to risk meeting a man, even though the pressure of being defined by their size is removed because of the specific nature of the agency. Sandy finds that she is constantly filled with anger at the distress caused to women. Young girls of eighteen ring her, in desperation, brainwashed by their peers or by parents, some of whom tell them they cannot have a boyfriend until they have lost weight. It is a hard selling job, she says, convincing them that their qualities as women and as partners are not defined by their weight, and she finds her job as much that of agony aunt as proprietor of a successful dating agency.

Feminists may raise doubts as to the dangers of voyeurism with a dating agency that offers fat women a chance to participate in seeking a partner in a way that is quite acceptable to those of 'normal' size. There is after all a difference in wanting a large woman as a companion and a partner, and the salacious titillation offered by the 'Roly-Poly Kissogram' girls. Sandy Millington is an astute woman who quickly learnt to recognize the occasional voyeur and to weed them out smartly. But they have been rare and she derives a quiet satisfaction from being able to offer a place where fat women can meet men, completely free from fear of rejection.

In the United States, NAAFA has a range of 'special interest groups' concerned with various aspects of being fat. One of these is the Fat Admirers' S.I.G., usually known as the FAs. Neil Dachis, a member of the group, writes:

A Fat Admirer is a person of either sex, any age, race or religion who has a certain psychological and physical orientation and composition which causes him/her to be sexually, sensually and psychologically aroused by and responsive to fat people of the same or opposite sex. More simply put, an FA is one who enjoys being with, looking at, thinking of, and being aroused by, a fat person. It is very important in defining what an FA is, to emphatically state what an FA is not. A Fat Admirer is *not* a deviant, pervert, a social outcast, a misfit, weirdo, or any other unfortunate label that may be placed on the FA. Those labels are sadly, but not surprisingly, used not just by some thin people, but some fat people as well.

What an indictment of mean-spirited, narrow-minded society — that not only is a fat person subject to pejorative labels, but so too is anyone who dares show a preference for or attraction to fat people. Dating agencies, like Sandy Millington's and NAAFA's Fat Admirers, are needed for several reasons: to give positive messages to the maligned fat; to counteract all those lonely hearts ads which say 'Slim attractive, etc, seeks . . .' or 'must be slim'; and finally, because some ordinary dating agencies will not accept fat people, especially fat women, on their books ('We wouldn't be able to place you, dear').[11]

A fifteen-year long study conducted by Dr Domeena Renshaw in Chicago has found that fat women are better lovers.[12] After treating one hundred and twenty-one women for eating and sexual disorders, the doctor concluded that women's sex lives are damaged more severely by excessive weight loss than by obesity. Women obsessed by thinness are so concerned with their weight and shape that they have fewer sexual fantasies and fewer encounters with men, she said. As their appetite for food dwindles so does their appetite for sex. Excessive weight gain rarely produces sexual problems, but anorexia and bulimia both diminish the sex drive — the thought of becoming pregnant is so abhorrent to such women that they cannot make peace with their bodies, reports Dr Renshaw.

Up till now I have talked about men's sexual evaluation of women and of women's evaluation of themselves in relation to men. What about lesbian relationships? There is a wistfully pervasive idea, mainly among straight women, that a lesbian relationship is automatically without sexual pressures or expectations 'because women are more caring of each other and understand each other's needs and feelings.' (I am referring to straight women to whom the idea of lesbian relationships is acceptable in principle at least.)

Talking to a group of gay women revealed that this gentle ideal is no more than that. Women looking for female lovers have in many respects the same criteria as men. They 'fancy' them in the same sort of way. Some lesbian social groups produce a newsletter which contains contact ads and a scan through a batch of these produces the same old yardsticks for acceptance. Women want 'slim woman to share . . .'; women describe themselves as slim, or thin. I found one or two advertisements from women apologising for the fact that they were 'plump' or stating that they were 'overweight but dieting'. As a feminist, I found this astonishing and disheartening, so convinced was I that female consciousness which included lesbianism would not set standards of looks or size in the partners they were seeking:

I do like a woman to have a nice body — that's very important to me. I like my own body and want to be able to admire the same sort of features in the body of the woman I go to bed with.

I do go for a certain type — every time — dark haired, slim, they must be slim. I get turned on by nice small firm buttocks.

I answered an ad in a gay magazine and thought I had found a partner. We wrote to each other and talked on the phone every night. She even said: 'Why didn't we find each other years ago?' I said how would we know until we met that it was right and she said: 'What difference can that make? We know each other. It's only seeing each other.' We met on Barnes Common in London and I knew that it wasn't going to work as soon as I saw the look in her eye — disappointment, distress, guilt. Years later, when we became friends, she told me that she didn't like fat women, but that she didn't know that until the day we met.

I fell in love with a woman, she was so beautiful, so gentle. She was kind, and warm and lovely and she started dropping hints that things could be pretty special between us. She invited me back to her flat one night and I made love to her. Then she said, very gently and sweetly — 'I'm not going to make love to you until you lose two stone. Then I will. It will be your reward.' I've never got over the humiliation.

At the first National Fat Women's Conference in March 1989, a group of lesbians talked about the problems of being fat and gay. They were doubly oppressed by society, they said, and oppressed by feminists for being fat. They felt buffeted between the gay and straight worlds. Straight people made the assumption that they were lesbian only because their fat prevented them from getting a man and regarded them as 'failed heterosexuals'. But the feminist ideals of women being just how they wanted to be had never existed, they said. Their fat was no more acceptable in the lesbian/feminist world because the same stringent rules applied — the pressure may not have been on looking good in a way that was sexually attractive to men, but women had their own codes of what constituted sexual attractiveness to each other. Being fat did not come into it. Feminists, they said bitterly, were just as obsessed with being thin, but they cloaked it under concern for health and fitness. Turning up on the scene with a good-looking woman carried just the same image-consciousness that rules the lives of hetero-sexual men and women. The only scenario that was different was where a woman was 'butch' and fat, and was fancied because of her strength and power, not usually by another large woman but by small, 'femme' women. These fat 'butch' lesbians obviously resented being wanted for their macho strength, but it is interesting to note that, as in the heterosexual game, it is the macho, beefy, big strong man elements that were acceptable. Never mind if the butch lesbian didn't want to feel like a man or play a man's role — that was the only guise under which fat lesbians were considered desirable. In America, fat lesbians have been working for acceptance as fat lesbians, just as in both Britain and America, fat women have tried to fight for the same acceptance.

The other point that emerged from the fat lesbians talking was the problem of lovemaking. In heterosexual sex the act is an anatomical fusion of two bodies. In lesbian lovemaking there are elements of activity and passivity; there is making love and being made love to. And the women who felt bad about their fat bodies found themselves in the age old female place of being the giver — they could make love to their partner, but could not easily accept being make love to, in case they repelled their partner, or from a conviction that it must be revolting to have to make love to their fat bodies. So they were constantly giving, and constantly deprived. It was clear that where lesbianism is a part of feminism, then feminists have let their sisters down badly.

FRIENDSHIPS

Do we as fat women suspect the motives of our friends? And have we any reason to do so? I think the answer must be yes, sometimes, on both counts. We are so often expected to be the providers and we take on this role unconsciously in a friendship because it is part of the persona many of us have developed as an apology and an offering, a sacrificial lamb for our sin of being fat. So we behave meekly like lambs. We allow our friends to put upon us, to use us, to drain us, while we ask for nothing back, except their friendship. We do not say, hey, you hurt me when you say that. We do not say, no, you cannot come to stay, I'm working too hard, I'm tired, or I've got other things I must do. We are afraid we will lose them. And it becomes circular again, because many of our friendships are based on these qualities which we lay before people — of being there as universal mother, provider, listener. We do not dare scream out — STOP — I have feelings and problems and I hurt too, and I want someone to talk to and I want YOU to listen to ME. We did not incorporate that into the initial contract when we started the friendship. We did not betray our wants and needs. And when we feel we would like to test the water, we fear it will be too cold. And we fear coldness. As long as our friends need us, come to us for comfort, rest their heads on our comfortable shoulders, we have warmth. We are needed. We are not rejected.

I had a friend once who was beautiful and conscious of her beauty. She would come over for the evening. I would go to her for supper. There was ease of conversation and laughter. But she seemed to avoid being with me at any kind of public gathering. Then one day we were both at the private view of an exhibition. I joined her as she moved round the gallery. As I reached her side she moved away. I followed her. She moved away again. Then she joined a group of people I did not know. I was puzzled, hurt, betrayed. Best ignore it, I thought. But I couldn't. So I rang her and said I felt that she did not want to be seen in public with me. She hesitated, then said, yes, I was right, she did not want the world at large to see that we were friends, not unless we were part of a group. She was ashamed, but unrepentant. She was part of the Beautiful Set. Together they regularly visited health farms and beauty parlours. It did not do her image any good to be seen on intimate terms with someone who had 'let herself go'. I ended the friendship. Fine, she said. As long as I understood that it was my problem.

On the other hand, a tested friendship, like my friend Gail's can be a harbour in storm when we are beset with censure and advice we don't want about our bodies. It is a treasure of great worth to be, as the cliché runs, 'accepted just as you are'. For fat women, those friends that they know they can trust utterly are especially precious and there are probably few that they feel completely at home with. And friendship is always being tested. The other day a friend I thought I was close to remarked that she had to exercise the most enormous willpower when she went to the fridge for anything to prevent herself from getting something out and eating it. Only that way, she said, was she able to maintain her weight. She really was very weak-willed by nature and fought tremendous battles every day. This told me two things: that the idea of being fat — even of putting on any weight at all — was anathema. And that the cause of this dreadful thing was, in her mind, indulgence and lack of will-power. There I sat, living testimony of the twin evils she fights daily. How can friends truly love you if they are spending a sizeable portion of their life fighting not to become like you? It feels like a diluted, conditional love again.

And do they use us, we wonder. Do they use us, consciously or otherwise, to offset their slimness, their control, their virtue, their ability to wear real clothes, not garments of limited choice bought by mail order or from Evans? Do we, in fact, boost their egos? From one letter:

I discovered recently that my so-called best friend wanted to go to parties and dances with me only because she reckoned that next to me she looked really attractive and the boys would fancy her. I am a size 20, she is a size 12. I am so hurt that I have not been out or seen anyone for over a month. I just keep thinking what a fool I have been to trust her.

Are we paranoically suspicious of our friends' motives? I don't think so, on the whole. The glorious thing is that when we discover the friends who genuinely love us just as we are, would love us the same if we put on another ten stones, they seem far more precious than friends acquired easily or casually. It is something like the test for dross and gold and when we find the gold, we recognize it.

MOTHERS

Mothers are rarely able to be indifferent to their daughters' size because to them it speaks such volumes about their own mother-love. My mother fed me, substituting food for the time she wanted to spend with me and could not because she was supporting my father in his business. She was torn between his needs and mine. His won. I doubted her loyalty but never her love. When I got fat, she must have known the cause. There is no history of fat in my family; all are minute Celts. But she needed to give me love so she went on giving me food. It is a very basic, mother-thing to do. And when I railed and shouted and cried that I was fat, that I was different she tried to soothe me by saying I was imagining it, that I wasn't fat, that I was 'just right' — it was the others who were too thin. And I didn't believe her, so though she tried to be my support, my ally, she unwittingly put herself in opposition to me by not acknowledging and understanding my pain.

The women who wrote, who shared their feelings and experiences with me, who talked about their lives and their pain, nearly all mentioned their mothers. None of the fat women who brought me their lives was indifferent or calm about her mother. Mothers figured large, important, whether alive or dead.

I didn't want to be like my mother, she was like a doll. She was slim and manicured and coiffed and perfect. And she wanted me to be the same. I didn't know I was setting out to get fat to spite her, but she was so distressed, that's what I must have done.

My mother wanted me to do well, to be brilliant at school, to go to university and to have a marvellous career because she didn't manage to. And I couldn't make it and I got tense and started eating to calm me down, and then I realized that my failure had left a great empty hole inside — which was my mother's disappointment in me. So I ate to fill it and I still do.

My mother says she'll help me lose weight. And then she comes to visit and she always brings food, it's as though she can't help it, and I can't resist it. It's as though that way she stops me controlling my own life because I can never say no to the food.

I was startled and delighted and relieved when one woman spoke to me of her experience regarding her mother's death:

I never got on with the old bag. But I was not prepared for her to go so suddenly. I think that I always thought some day when we're both old and mellow we would make our peace. But there was never a chance. And since then I have just got fatter and fatter. I'm filling some space, I know that, but I don't know how or why.

Carol Lopacich was cut out of her mother's multi-million dollar will because she was fat. During her childhood, Lopacich was subjected to daily weigh-ins and lectures. She ran away from home and was sent to boarding school. Her mother told friends she didn't have a daughter. When Carol Lopacich called her mother to say that she was married, her mother's first question was 'What do you weigh?' When Lopacich said she was still fat, her mother said she couldn't see her because she was entertaining guests. When Lopacich finally attempted to win her mother's approval by losing 200 lb it was too late — her mother was too ill to recognise her and died shortly after.

It prompted me to think about my own mother's death in 1985. I had not made the connection before, but since that time I have put on more weight than at any other time in my life. And it has been the only period of my life that I have been unable to lose it. My mother's death, which was sudden and premature, left so much unfinished business. Most of all it left an emptiness that I was quite unprepared for and a desolation that is like nothing else has ever been.

The mother/daughter relationship is perhaps more complex than any other. There are no absolute rules regarding the link between our fatness and our relationship with our mothers. While my mother fed me and I grew fat, my friend's experience was completely different.

Jennifer's mother was obsessed with her weight and with her children's. She continually put Jennifer on diets, even though she was not fat, and chastised her for eating. Reaching out to the dish of potatoes on the table she would be met by a warning 'Now, now Jennifer . . .' She would take her into clothes shops, appealing to assistants for sympathy. 'Look at her', she would say. 'What can you do with her?' Jennifer dieted for her mother, wanting to please her, believing that she was right. And her brother just grew fat. Now, with a metabolism in ruins after a lifetime of dieting and gaining, Jennifer is middle-aged and fat, and so is her brother. Jennifer reflects grimly on life with a mother who prized slimness and tried so hard to impose it on her children. 'What did she end up with after all her pains? says Jennifer. 'Two fat children.'

Dr George Blackburn, who helped developed Optifast and Slimfast was quoted as saying: 'If there is no evidence of illness or cosmetic or psychological problems resulting from excess body weight, there is no reason to diet . . . Parents with obese children should lay off.'

From NAAFA Newsletter, February 1992

It isn't only mothers. One man said to his three-year old daughter, 'Don't eat all those biscuits or you'll get fat and Daddy won't love you any more.' A friend, overhearing this, asked the man what he would have said to a son. He replied: 'I'd say don't eat all those biscuits because you'll get fat and you won't be able to play football.' The friend suggested he start saving for the fees to pay for treatment for his daughter's future eating disorder, the seeds of which he had just sown.

I know from my own daughters' responses that children and adolescents are deeply influenced by advertising. They take television commericals and magazine advertisements quite literally and it is here that we have a great responsibility as mothers. We need to make our children highly aware of the pressures within our culture and to teach them that being beautiful and thin does not lead to health and happiness. There are enough media stars who conform to our cultural image and who have drug, divorce, alcohol or other health problems for us to be able to use them as an illustration that looking like that does not lead to a better life.

I also believe we have a responsibility to give our children a positive role model in ourselves, and this is not easy if we have not come to terms with our own fatness. But it is essential, even if we do it by deceit of some kind, not to denigrate our bodies and make our daughters feel that the media are right — this is something to be avoided at all costs because look how badly Mum feels about it. They are going to be exposed to so many negative evaluations about fatness that we have to provide positive images to counteract these.

One study of American girls aged nine to eighteen found that they all feared being fat. Fifty per cent of the nine year olds had already been put on diets. Nearly 90 per cent of the seventeen year olds dieted regularly. They *all* believed that dieting was the normal way to eat.[13] Alice Ansfield, editor of the American magazine for fat acceptance, *Radiance,* stated in an editorial: 'Greater numbers of kids are throwing up their food or are starving themselves in their desperation to be thin. I've heard of some high school parties where girls are admitted only after weighing in.'[14]

I also believe that we should avoid falling into the easy trap of sympathising with the plight of a fat child. It is almost automatic, especially if we are identifying with her pain, because we too were once fat children. But if our daughters hear our message of sympathy the alarm bells about being fat will be set off again. Better to emphasize the good points of a fat child, give them a positive sense of identity regardless of body size.

I heard a woman talk of how, when she was a teenager, her mother would lie in bed at night thinking of the disgrace of having a fat daughter. Some nights the mother would jump out of bed, run to her daughter's room, wake her up, tear off her nightgown, stand her in front of a mirror, and scream at her that she was a disgusting child who was a disgrace to the family.

Russell F. Williams speaking at NAAFA Media Image Rally, 1989

We have to tread a fine line with our own children, especially if we are mothers of daughters. A woman who has lived a life of fat misery can produce anorexia in her daughter in her desire for the girl not to suffer as she has. We can make our daughters too conscious of their bodies and of their eating patterns by being over anxious when we think they are eating too much or the wrong food. And we also have to balance the pressure they are under from their peers to be thin; not slim, not average, but thin. As fat mothers we walk a tightrope.

Mothers. They are books and books in themselves. It is impossible to allocate a section of a book to the mother/daughter relationship. But being fat is not an individual solitary state. Our fatness was not created by ourselves but by the combination of influences outside ourselves. We may become fat because of emotional deprivation, or because of some kind of parental influence. Our being fat affects our relationships with our parents, our children, our friends and our lovers. It has ramifications that reach through the whole of our lives and touch the way we interact with others and they with us.

5

The tyranny of fashion

It is a powerful statement about current attitudes to body size that our word 'obese' actually derives from the Latin word *obesus* meaning 'eaten up' or 'lean'. What happened in the translation reflects something of the cultural differences regarding fatness around the world. Here, in affluent Western society it is unequivocally uncompromising. Obese, somehow an unpleasantly onomatopoeic word, is a two-syllabled condemnation of a socially despised state. Physicians deliberately divide weight into several categories: underweight, normal weight, overweight, obese, grossly obese, morbidly obese. How many of us, while honestly admitting to being overweight (though by whose definition?) could equally unflinchingly describe ourselves as obese? It is not a matter of choosing euphemisms, overweight is a descriptive, definitive word; obese carries all the ugliness attributed to the condition of being fat.

Turn the coin over and we find the ideal state for the modern woman — thinness. 'You cannot be too rich or too thin,' said the Duchess of Windsor in the 1930s, and our culture sees no reason to argue with that half a century later. Yet the word 'thin' used to have considerable negative connotations, to be associated with meanness, spite, to be ungenerous, unyielding. In Victorian times we read in novels of the thin spinster with the pince-nez, suggesting a body unrounded by physical love or childbearing or suckling. Thin means meagre; in fact the French word is *maigre* and to slim in French is *maigrir* — to become meagre! Thin on the ground, to have a thin time — these colloquialisms are used to indicate pretty bleak states; the dictionary uses words like wretched and uncomfortable.

Roget's Thesaurus gives us no suggestion of the desirability of being thin. Its list of adjectives following the word 'thin' are enough to arouse pity for the creatures if we did not know better: 'meagre, skinny, bony, cadaverous, fleshless, skin-and-bone, skeletal, raw-boned, haggard, gaunt, drawn, lantern-jawed, hatchet-faced, twiggy, spindly, spindle-shanked, spidery, undersized, weedy, scrawny, scraggy, consumptive, emaciated, shrivelled, pinched, peaky'. And the verb 'to make thin' is defined as 'contract, compress, pinch, nip'. This, then, is what women are encouraged to seek and achieve for their bodies and for which they are socially outcast if they do not attain the meagre state.

The development of language is a curious phenomenon. In hot, Mediterranean countries where the weather and lifestyle encourage the enjoyment of food and sensual pleasures, the androgynous figure had no place until the British and American move towards extreme thinness which began in the 1960s. Now, in Italy, where plumpness was once considered essentially female, a fat woman is insulted by the use of the word *balena,* meaning whale. Whales have always been used in disparaging comparison with large womansize — 'like a beached whale', 'whale blubber', 'Moby Dick'. But now the world has finally recognized the grace and beauty of these creatures and a beached whale is considered a creature to be loved, rescued, cared for and restored. With the world's attention focused on the plight of these disappearing beasts we are realizing what we have so nearly lost and how much poorer we would be without the whales. It is hardly appropriate to use *balena* as a term of abuse.

It is a sensitive subject, the use of descriptive words for the woman who in the eyes of society is too big. Feminists are trying to reclaim the word 'fat' but it has had such violently negative associations for so long that it is difficult for many women to own to being fat. It carries a sense of shame and degradation, memories of childhood taunts: 'fatty, fatso'. The substance itself is not a palatable one for most people, who do not want fat on their meat, or the greasy, white substance that solidifies on top of cold gravy. In addition to a certain aesthetic repugnance, we now have the knowledge about the badness of animal fat, the cholesterol-producing, artery-clogging, creeping death hastener. So our associations with the word fat are all negative, with no positive overtones to be found in the *Thesaurus* which lists, with a certain amount of relish it seems to me; 'fat person — tub, dumpling, mound of flesh, tub of lard, lard-lump, hulk, Bunter, Falstaff'.

Yet if we go back to the beautiful, elegant language of the King James Bible, we find both the word fat and its attributes praised and celebrated. In the wonderful psalm of harvest thanksgiving, where the folds are full of sheep and the valleys stand so thick with corn that they shall laugh and sing, the psalmist says: 'Thou crownest the year with thy goodness and thy clouds drop fatness.' A beautiful, direct association between good and beauty and plenty and rejoicing.

In the earliest times mankind's greatest preoccupation was staying alive which included finding enough food. Fatness was an unattainable ideal — a far-off symbol of prosperity. But fertility was worshipped and the earliest prehistoric symbols were figures of clay and terracotta made several thousand years BC. These statues included the Venus of Willendorf, dated at around 30,000 BC and considered to be the very oldest symbol of fertility and of the Goddess. Typically the figures are large-breasted with swelling bellies, large thighs and bottoms. These sculptures represented the beginnings of Goddess worship and the recognition by men of female power. The image of this large and bountiful woman held sway for many centuries, she was the mother of the Earth and of all mankind and myths and rituals sprang from beliefs that her fertility came from within herself, without the help of an external male. It was the reign of the matriarch.

The rise of feminism in the 1970s brought with it a rejection of the notion of a male God and a return to the ancient rituals of Goddess worship. The goddess symbols painted and sculpted today are similar to those prehistoric ones with minimal attention given to head or lower legs. I have one in my study, made for me by a friend. The figure stands on her thighs, her belly and breasts are huge, her head is a symbolic apple. I am intrigued and amused by most people's reactions to her — they think she is grotesque, though that may be because her sexual organs are freely and frankly depicted.

Feminists may talk about the Goddess but do they really embrace all that she stands for? I think most do not. Female power and a matriarchal society, the response to too many centuries of male oppression, maybe. But the generous fertile hugeness of the Goddess? I feel it is significant of the feminists' rejection of this aspect that it is only very recently in Britain that we have seen the formation of fat women's groups and their brave emergence into thin society. Some groups want to reclaim the word 'fat', just as the National Association for the Advancement of Fat Acceptance has done in America.

I believe strongly that we have been deluded into believing that feminists have taken up the cause of the fat woman, have helped her to accept her size and the positive symbolism associated with her body. The book *Fat is a Feminist Issue*[1] by Susie Orbach has been misunderstood by many women. The book is not about allowing yourself the freedom to be fat in a male-dominated, media-oriented thin society. The shout-line on the cover leaps out challengingly in red: 'How to lose weight permanently without dieting'. The basis for this book is the problem of compulsive eating and it is a book for anorexics, bulimics and women who feel out of control around food. Orbach states that: 'Compulsive eating is an individual protest against the inequality of the sexes.'

This is a facile over-simplification of the complex motives behind compulsive eating. There are a number of men who eat — or drink — compulsively, too, the difference being that it is more socially acceptable for a man to be fat (large, solid, weighty, reassuring, authoritative). Compulsive eating is *one* of a great many reasons for becoming fat, but Orbach's premise is overstating the case. She postulates — and she is not the only one — that we invest our power in our fat, that once we uncover and understand our own individual motivations for being fat, we can re-invest that power in ourselves, and in learning to love food and use it appropriately we will only eat what our bodies need.

For a certain type of fat woman this is undoubtedly so — but experience shows that this woman is the one who swings from one end to the other of the anorexic-overweight scale with bulimia in between. In addition, Orbach's method of encouraging women to form self-help therapy groups is probably even more effective than her psychology, as the success of Weight Watchers and other similar clubs has proved. The effect of group dynamics is powerful when there is a fusion of people with the same problems, the same fears, feelings and aspirations.

But Orbach is no more on the side of fat women than is the patriarchal society she claims to reject. In fact, she colludes with its expectations of women: 'We know that every woman wants to be thin. Our images of womanhood are almost synonymous with thinness.'

I would not find that statement out of place in a beauty article in *Vogue* but I find it extraordinarily narrow-minded in a feminist of Orbach's standing. It is true that most women would like to lose some weight[2] but what makes Orbach assume that we all want to be thin? I don't; I would simply like to be less fat — a great deal different from thin.

I feel I need to say something at this point about the whole question of feminism and fatness because there is a great deal of misunderstanding around this issue. There *are* feminists who are working hard to end fat oppression as they have worked to end other kinds of oppression; Vivian Mayer, who has done so much pioneering work in this field and who contributed to *Shadow on a Tightrope,* a marvellous collection of fat women's writings,[3] is one such person. In fact, all the women who have written for that book are feminists but many of them speak of the pain of being rejected by the one group they thought they could trust — other feminists. In one of the essays in the collection, *The Fat Illusion,* Vivian Mayer says: 'In gatherings of the highest revolutionary spirit you will see right-on feminists drinking cans of diet soda to avoid being fat ... Aside from superficial awareness that fat women are oppressed by looksism, radical women still see fat as a personal sickness: abnormal, undesirable, lamentable and curable.' Another essay, *Some Thoughts on Fat* by Joan Dickenson, examines the assumption that however it is achieved, thinness is still desirable. 'Why don't we try to change society's image of beauty on the one hand, and arm fat women in confidence and pride on the other? We do neither. Instead we try to teach women *not* to be fat! Isn't this like telling a rape victim to relax and enjoy it?' However much feminists — or anyone else — may feel like protesting at such a powerful analogy, their protest will come from a sense of discomfort that there is truth in it. Fat *is* a problem, writes Joan Dickenson, but the question is *whose* problem? She too feels let down by

Orbach: 'By stating that each woman can solve it for herself, Orbach implies . . . that the problem is ours. Thinness is best, she says . . . it is a woman's duty to try for it and therefore it is her fault if she fails. Blame the victim.'

Susie Orbach represents the majority of women, and that includes committed feminists, by taking as her thesis the desirability of thinness. Find out what your fat is doing for you and then you can lose it, is her message. She herself was 'afraid' of being thin; once that was sorted out she had no more obstacles to overcome on the way to this desirable state. My inability to feel that Orbach and I are working in the same field comes from a sense of alienation from her, a difficulty in feeling a rapport with someone who is telling me, in effect, that I am *not* acceptable, stable, whole, as a fat woman. I am also cynical — a book whose subtitle is 'How to Lose Weight Permanently Without Dieting' could not have been written by a woman who wants to change the world's antipathy towards fat people.

I am, I realize, extremely angry at the myth that feminists are our allies. I feel betrayed, conned, let down, deserted. Feminists are powerful — they have *claimed* this power through as many means as they could. When they believe in something they can be radical to the point of violence, especially if they believe in militancy. Their voices are loud — they do not see themselves as weak, nor do they accept scapegoating. There *are* feminists fighting the battle against fat oppression but still they are in the minority. Why is this?

Dale Spender, writer, activist and a leader amongst feminists says: 'Being fat is never acceptable. Women comment about it as much as men. Feminists are not immune. I'm certainly not. You watch women, even the fiercest, most politically ideologically correct, summing up other women when they see them running to flab. You see the signs as they say, "She's overweight, poor old thing, thank goodness I'm thinner than she is".'

Sally Cline, another feminist activist, quotes Dale Spender's admission in her own book about women and food, *Just Desserts*.[4] Dale, she says, is an extremely thin woman whose weight rarely rises above 7½ stones (105lb), and who became anorexic at the age of 43. Anorexia, incidentally, is not the sole province of young girls and women with an unformed sense of their own identity — it occurs, though less frequently, in mature women who have proved themselves in the eyes of the world, professionally or otherwise. Like Dale Spender, whose excellent work as a writer is fully recognized.

A great deal of *Just Desserts* is autobiographical, an interesting account of the part played by food in a Jewish family. The last chapter, though, attempts to examine the way in which women — feminists — oppress fat women. Sally Cline uses herself and her own prejudice as an example of this. She describes how, in a hospital clinic, she heard a mellow, melodic voice asking her for her autograph. She describes her feeling of pride and pleasure as she looked around for the source of the voice, and her disappointment when she saw the woman who had spoken: 'a sort of cloth pyramid earnestly flapping a paperback in my direction'. Sally Cline says she felt let down 'as if the praise of a fat woman was somehow not as legitimate as the praise of a thin woman or of a man'. In the ensuing conversation between the two women, Trudie, the fat admirer of Sally Cline's work, confided what it felt like to be fat, shared with Sally the pain, rejection and humiliation. This made Sally extremely uncomfortable and caused her to question the legitimacy of her feelings about her own body — at about 9½ stones (132lb) she describes herself as 'flabby . . . lumbering . . . trying to improve my life chances by subduing my recalcitrant flesh'.

She invited Trudie to visit her at home, to talk more and to examine her own reactions to this very large woman.

Cline struggled with her own ideology concerning the oppression of minority groups, an ideology that condemned the evils of the oppression and victimisation of women, lesbians, Jews and those with disabilities. She admits to having felt miserable, put down and patronised, overlooked and discriminated against. But she had fought the oppression, feeling 'righteous' she says, and she had found that fight elating. Yet with her feminist and political beliefs about human rights, she confesses that she sat opposite Trudie 'playing the worthy feminist author, drawing her out, wondering secretly how she could bear to look like that, smirking slyly at my own slim legs, thankful the scales only registered nine and a half stone today'.

With complete frankness, Sally Cline shows herself in an unfavourable light. She records her reactions to Trudie — why was she eating the bun Sally had offered her?; surely she shouldn't be putting jam on it; how does she ever find anything decent to wear?; at some level it must be her own fault; what about walking about naked — wasn't she ashamed? She admits to irritation at Trudie spilling over the chair she was sitting in, and later when she had difficulty fastening the car safety belt.

I am ambivalent about Sally Cline's attempt to examine fat oppression and to admit to it herself. At one level I know I should admire her frankness and I think at some level of my consciousness I do. But another part of me is unable to understand how a feminist — a woman on the side of women, someone who has fought for other hated and oppressed groups — can denigrate, however unwillingly, another woman simply because she is fat. And with what may seem like the deepest cynicism, I question Sally Cline's motive for telling Trudie's story, simply because she questions it herself: 'How can I write this and feel unashamed or good about myself knowing that Trudie will suffer (again) as she reads it . . . How can I print these words and know that Trudie, a sad, fat, betrayed woman trusted me enough as a sister, a feminist, to tell me all the things that have hurt her because she is fat . . . trusted me to be on her side . . . when she is surrounded by other people's hatred of her flesh?'

Sally Cline's explanation is that Trudie's story needed to be told in order to expose the horrors of fat oppression, including the author's own. But could she not have disguised this woman and their encounter in such a way that Trudie need not have read the account and felt betrayed? It could have been done, the points made just as forcefully; for the pain and shame experienced by fat women makes its sharing an intimacy, rarely risked. For this reason all the accounts and identities trusted to me by fat women and used in this book have been disguised. I realize that my anger at this author's betrayal of a fat woman's trust comes from my own and from the collective experience of being betrayed by those whom we thought valued us, not in spite of our fat but without even labelling us as such. These people are few in the lives of many fat women and most will resonate with the memory of having been let down, at least once in such a way. Sally Cline says she knows that it is her fat-hatred she weighs when she stands on the scales and it is that hatred that she sustains if she loses a few pounds. And she admits that while there is no such thing as a fat frame of mind, only differently sized people, society's persistent anti-fat propaganda prevents most of us from recognizing this. 'Me included' she says.

And this is the point. Sally Cline shows us that feminists, as a group are no different from anyone else in their prejudice.

So, how can we reclaim the Goddess if our 'images of womanhood are almost synonymous with thinness'? Whose images and what womanhood? As a very large woman myself I am well aware that society as a whole and individuals within it may despise me for my size from an aesthetic and moral standpoint. I also know that there are very many men, women and children who enjoy the voluptuousness of being hugged and held by a large, soft woman. It may sound paradoxical, but when I hug thin friends I feel I cannot get very close to them because there is nothing substantial to hold in my arms, no flesh to meet and blend with. And a couple of sharp, pointed pelvic bones digging in when you get close to a thin person HURTS!

I love the Goddess Earth Mother image, the fecund look of full breasts, curving hips and padded bottoms, undulating and flowing in undisciplined forms. I love the fullness of flesh under loose garments and the sight of plump arms holding a baby to a breast that is overflowing in every sense. I enjoy the almost incandescent glow of Renoir's fat women, the Renaissance Madonnas, large, stately opera singers and of course Rembrandt and Rubens. It gives me pleasure to see black women whose cultures have not dictated that they lose their glowing, naturally bountiful shapes.

Given absolute choice, forced to respond with total honesty, I look back at photographs, and in my memories, to the different images of myself at various weights and stages of my life, and I can say that I would not like to be thin. As a teenager I suffered as all teenagers do with the curse of being 'different' but with adult experience and perception I am not bound by those chains of conformity. It is not comfortable to be as heavy as I am and instinctively I do not feel at home in this body as it is now. The image that leaps out, looking back down the years is of a glowing, radiant woman with a new baby — myself with my second child. She is large, this woman, and her body suggests a relaxed ease with itself, a recognition that body and spirit are well reconciled. This woman is clearly the right weight for her. I remember how she felt, energetic, agile, wearing

Indian cotton voile dresses not because they were the only clothes available for her size but because she loved them and felt they matched the image she had of herself. Confident, not afraid because she did not fit in with social expectations. Yet this woman, myself at twenty-eight, weighed thirteen stones (185lb), overweight by social and medical definition, and only 5'4" in height. That is how I would choose to be again.

There are metabolic and psychological reasons why I have not remained at my ideal weight and they are something I have to work out for myself. But I am defying the school of psychological thought which says that by wishing to be thirteen stones — therefore 'grossly overweight' — I am refusing to face up to something which I wish to 'contain' in my layers of fat. I repudiate that and having done so I will attempt to articulate my own reasons for disagreeing with the bald Orbach pronouncement that every woman wants to be thin.

First, I am a sensual person and I cannot equate thinness with sensuality. I like being told I am cuddly. I like the acknowledgement of my flesh. I enjoy the visible, tangible symbols of fertility — the large breasts, round belly and curved hips. I feel like an Earth Mother and that is the way I want to feel.

Psychologically it is not in my nature to conform. There is an apparent paradox here because I have stated in several places in this book that the stigma of not conforming leads to great pain. But my pain — and it is an individual thing for each fat woman — comes from being stigmatised at the weight I am now. I did not feel outcast when I was thirteen stones (185lb) because I was happy with myself. And somewhere in there is the crux of the understanding of a fat woman's feelings about herself. We are told that we must learn to love ourselves, accept ourselves the way we are. But we all carry inside ourselves an image of how we want to be. For many women this *is* a longing to be slim. But not for all — which is why some women are suicidally unhappy at my ideal weight while others are able to live with and love themselves at fifteen (210), sixteen (225), seventeen stones (240lb) — though they are rare, such is the potency of social pressure. It is just too facile to say that we must love ourselves when we are being battered on all sides to change, and unlike black or disabled people we are made to feel we have the means of doing so. If we can try to separate our individual feelings about size from the desperation to be 'normal' and therefore acceptable, we may find that for a multitude of different reasons, being thin would not suit us.

For me the idea of being thin is psychologically threatening. It carries associations of anonymity, facelessness. Just as many anorexics seek to recreate their childhood body in an attempt to escape their womanhood, either to avoid responsibility for their lives, to avoid their sexuality or to return to the state when they were pleasing to their fathers, so I find the idea of a return to childhood a frightening one as my childhood was full of insecurities. I was a powerless child in the face of adults in conflict, who placed upon my shoulders burdens they were unable to carry. For me a thin body recalls that helpless, powerless frightened state.

Every woman who is thin has the acceptance of the world we live in and for that reason alone the notion of thinness is a very seductive one. But I have two close friends who are thin, beautifully, acceptably thin. Yet one of them wears padded bras to feminise her androgynous figure — she swears she has discovered the only shop left in London that still stocks them! And the other one tells me how self-conscious she is if she ever strips in front of anyone, exposing her almost non-existent breasts. 'I can understand how painful it must be to be fat and to hate it,' she told me.

'I wouldn't change places with you. But sometimes I feel that your shape means that you are more of a woman than I am.'

I was invited several years ago to a feminist meeting to hear a group of performers, The Spare Tyre Theatre Company. Five talented women who performed sketches and sang — songs they had written themselves about eating, weight and food, sketches that did not seem appropriate for the shape and size of the members of this group. And why, I wondered, were they calling themselves 'Spare Tyre'? I stayed behind afterwards to talk to them. They were responsive and friendly and answered my puzzled questions. They did have weight problems, they assured me. They had been compulsive eaters and had formed self-help therapy groups based on *Fat is a Feminist Issue*. They were kind, wanting to help in any way they could. They gave me a tape of their songs. I liked them. But I asked them why they considered they had such a problem that they needed to devote their lives to writing songs and sketches about fatness. One of them said to me (how often have fat women heard this one): 'I used to be just like you.' They were warm and generous, these women, with none of the smugness often found in the 'I have succeeded in controlling my weight, why can't you?' type of formerly fat women. And they were talented and funny and I have, since that first meeting, found in them real support for fat women.

And this is the point. It is important to separate these two very disparate groups of women — the fat women, who are the inspiration and motivation for writing this book, and the 'thin-fat' women — an expression coined by Hilde Bruch for those who have had an eating disorder, anorexia, bulimia or compulsive eating. They are different. The thin-fat women will always be preoccupied with weight and the power of food, but they have lost whatever weight they had. Many of them never became at all overweight, though they had difficulties with food. Their psychological and emotional states do not resemble those of the women who have dieted and gained, or just gained. Many of us have not had what doctors would classify as an eating disorder and that is what singles us out as being unworthy of help. We have become fat through our own fault, following the devices and desires of our own hearts — why is it that when talking about fat the language of sin so often creeps in?

To quote Professor Cary Cooper of Manchester University: 'What you need to do is make up some fancy Latin name for overweight. Make it nice and complicated with the same important-sounding ring as anorexia nervosa and then they'll take it seriously.'[5]

It can be alienating to discover a group of non-fat women calling themselves Spare Tyre and it can be confusing for a fat woman to see these extremely slim women in performance, when it is obvious that they do not share the same problem. We see their thin bodies and we realize that we cannot share the same kind of pain. 'Thin-fat' women are those who have lost weight but still perceive themselves as fat. Or they may never have gained at all, through controlling their size by purging and vomiting. Nevertheless they carry the image of fatness as a reality from which they have escaped or a spectre waiting to claim them if they should relax.

A few years ago I went to some meetings of the Overeaters Anonymous group. I had met one or two of the members and found their encouragement an incentive and far more sensitively directed (I felt) than the Weight Watchers type of slimming club. When I arrived at the first meeting I was dismayed to find I was the only fat woman in the room, the only one with any kind of weight problem at all. The meeting is run on the same lines as Alcoholics Anonymous: each person says 'My name is . . . and I am a compulsive eater.' It sounded bizarre — this group of slim women talking about the way food controlled their lives and talking about their bodies as though they were fat. I told them I could not identify with them as my problems were not the same as theirs. They were in the grip of abnormal eating patterns. Belinda, thin as a reed, described how she went to the bakery first thing every morning and bought two fresh, crusty loaves which she took back to the house she shared. She sliced them and covered them with butter and apricot jam. If anyone else living in the house came into the kitchen during this ritual she said she was expecting friends for breakfast. 'It was ridiculous,' she said. 'It was obvious I was going to eat them myself.' And she did, then immediately went to the lavatory and vomited till the last remnants were gone. Then there was Teresa who took one hundred laxatives a day and ate 'everything in sight. If there was nothing else in the house I would eat raw, hard pulses out of their jars.' But Teresa was tall, blonde and very thin with a kind of feline grace.

Certainly these women had problems and needed the support of a group which would understand and not condemn. But the kind of struggles they were having all homed in on the same Orbach philosophical starting point: 'We know that all women want to be thin.' And damage their minds and bodies they may have done, but these women had made it. The image they presented as they walked down the street was one of social normality. Their 'sins' could be kept secret.

I feel that it is important that fat and thin-fat women recognize these differences. It is hard to listen to women talking about food and weight problems when they have no visible signs of this, and the fat woman may feel 'What does she know about it?' It is equally important to understand that any woman who has been unhappy or psychologically disturbed because of her body image, due to the pressures on women to reach a socially-constructed idea of perfection, is an ally though she experiences her pain in a different way.

Many political feminists have rejected the symbols of femininity, and espoused male dress and the androgynous shape, while goddess-worshipping. Before the advent of the male gods, there was no doubt that the women deities ruled unchallenged. Goethe refers to the *Ewig-Weibliche* – the Eternal-Womanly, symbol of beauty, bringer of prosperity, good fortune. Eternal-Womanly appeared in many guises while she reigned but all her images are fat ones. In her book *The Moon and the Virgin*, Nor Hall talks of the matriarchal goddesses as 'life abundant, radiating from her mid-region ... Sanctity of the body, body inviolate, fused with the earth, this Mother is the Hill itself. She is a mountainous mass of earth ...'[6]

These are huge women, powerfully abundant. Too frightening in their power to be accepted. Yet still they exert an irresistible fascination. I live in Glastonbury, centre of myth and awakener of primitive instincts. There is the Tor, a huge prehistoric mound, considered the place of the Goddess. Pilgrimages are made all year round to climb the Tor, to be close to something indefinable, ancient and, few people would deny it, essentially female. The Tor is often likened to a huge breast and when people reach the top they lie down and embrace its vastness, to be at one with the great Mother. By no coincidence the town is full of shops where you can buy statues of women, goddesses, as full, as huge and as fecund as any from primitive art. Glastonbury Tor strikes some ancient memory that our civilization has lost something crucial in its relentless pursuit of a false ideal – that of ascetic control of the body.

The ancient Greeks were having none of this, of course. With their striving for physical and spiritual harmony they brought in the notion of aesthetic perfection and that did not embrace fatness. Anything that overflowed was out –

Photographer Patricia Schwarz of San Francisco was recently awarded the 1989 Ruttenberg Foundation Award, a prestigious award that honors fine art portrait photography. One Ruttenberg is awarded each year by the Friends of Photography, an internationally known organization founded by photographer Ansel Adams.

'For a jury of one to select a "winner" out of several thousand slides by 250 photographers isn't easy. How to choose one fine apple compared to an orange, a guava, a basket of delicious cherries and pears? Collage, maybe? Color or black and white? Handpainted silver prints? Beaches? Nicaragua? Tennessee backwoods? Bedrooms? The homeless in American streets?

'Somehow, the 250 names were narrowed down to a list of nineteen finalists, who were then invited to submit prints on paper. All did.

'I managed then to select four images from four photographers – Steve Cagan's unforgettable Central American "Little Boy with Stringed Instrument" (my titles); Patty Baldwin Detzel's compassionate magistral color print of her aged "Grandmother", Marna Clark's beautifully seen and printed black and white "Pubescent Girl;" and Patricia Schwarz' "Fat Lady."

'My final selection as winner of the Ruttenberg Fellowship Award was Patricia Schwarz, for her boldly colorful, boldly obese unclothed woman.

'Don't laugh, Schwarz doesn't. She gives us here an image of surprising beauty and shocking originality. Fat ladies are supposed to be laughed at, right? Or ignored. Or pitied. Schwarz presents hers most seriously, in a pose as formal and classic as a nude by Ingres.

'And it ain't funny. It's beautiful. It's daringly fresh. It makes us rethink both our graphic and our sexual stereotypes. It may become, I think, a classic in the collections and history of photography.'

Lou Stoumen, Juror 1989 Ruttenberg Foundation Fellowship

strict boundaries were in. Since then, appreciation of the large female body has re-occurred at times in Western culture and art; roundness and plumpness has been encouraged and valued according to changing notions of fashion and beauty. Bosoms and hips flowed and curved during the eighteenth and much of the nineteenth centuries, and the emphasis was on shape rather than size.

The insanity really started with the Victorian wasp waists. The idea behind this was to attain the true hour-glass shape — defined bosom and hips and non-existent middle. Women were laced into their corsets so tightly that they could not breathe — this is why Victorian women were so given to fainting and 'the vapours' and seen as rather feminine and delicate, while in reality their internal organs were being crushed and their lives shortened. The most ambitiously fashionable women went a stage further — the impediment to an even smaller waist was their lower rib on either side, so with the recent development of anaesthesia they underwent operations to remove these offending objects, thus allowing their stays to be laced even more tightly. We might exclaim with horror at such madness, but we should remember that we have not progressed; a hundred years later we have all manner of surgical procedures to remove fat and to ensure that we do not process and digest our food. We may not have the same risks of inadequate antisepsis, or anaesthetics, but women still consent to life-threatening operations in the name of beauty and vanity.

Edwardian women tended to be buxom and from the exasperated writings of a certain Dr Heckel in 1911, their choice of shape showed no obsessive desires for thinness. It was the era of the décolleté and women wanted to show off their well-covered upper breasts and cleavage. Heckel wrote:

One must mention here that aesthetic errors of a worldly nature to which all women submit, may make them want to stay obese for reasons of fashionable appearance. It is beyond doubt that in order to have an impressive décolleté each woman feels herself duty bound to be fat around the neck, over the clavicle and in her breasts. Now it happens that fat accumulates with greatest difficulty in these places and one can be sure, even without examining such a woman, that the abdomen and the hips and the lower members are hopelessly fat. As to the treatment, one cannot obtain weight reduction of the abdomen without the woman sacrificing in her spirits the upper part of her body. To her it is a true sacrifice because she gives up what the world considers beautiful.[7]

It is interesting to note the parallels with two periods in modern history when women fought to gain equal rights. In the 1920s, with the rise of the suffrage movement, the fashion was for cropped hair, flat (bound) breasts and a slim, androgynous shape. With the second wave of the Women's Movement in the early 1970s, some women sought a way of disowning their femininity. Bra-burning was a symbolic, collective metaphor for emancipation. And transvestism re-occurred, this time bringing along a new wave of women — the radical feminists and political lesbians who professed only to feel comfortable in men's clothes and with the shortest possible hair. Yet nobody would call a woman in a man's suit a transvestite, and male evening clothes have been given the seal of approval by current fashion trends.

As women continue the fight for equality they also continue to take on outwardly masculine identity, aided by fashion designers. A magazine article discusses the manufacture of frankly male clothes for women. The writer tells us of a 'male undershirt for women', that Calvin Klein is releasing 'bikinis and tanks cut like a man's briefs and undershirts' and that American women are 'dressing themselves all the way down to the skin in menswear'.

While women may feel this is a necessary move — that in order to be considered equal with men they have to show themselves to be the *same* as men — it puts the fat woman's body even further outside the range of acceptability. You cannot wear women's clothes designed for men if you have breasts, and hips and fecund-looking bellies.

Yet during the Second World War women were of necessity recognized as equals and by all accounts thrived on it. It appears that where we do not have to clamour for equality we revert to choosing to display our femininity — by feeling free to be full-breasted and curvaceous. I believe that war, with its rationing and privations and its huge loss of life, may arouse in the collective unconscious the instinct to procreate and to feed the body. History has always reflected that where fertility and the need for food were paramount, the images of women also reflected those priorities. There was no place for thinness.

Leanness is not a disadvantage to men ... But as regards the fair sex, it is a dreadful evil, for with them BEAUTY is more than LIFE, and BEAUTY consists especially in the rounded limb and the graceful curve. The best dressmaker in the world cannot conceal certain 'absences' or disguise certain angles ...

Brillat-Savarin, French gourmet philosopher in the chapter 'Leanness and its cure' from his book *Handbook of Dining*, 1825

I would like at this point to challenge Arthur Marwick, the historian, whose book *Beauty in History*[8] may be destined to become a classic. Marwick and I start from opposite corners of the ring with his contention that beauty is universal and not, as is said, in the eye of the beholder.

Marwick states that cultures which value fatness are cultures which value wealth and status above human beauty. While this may be true of the Aga Khan, who received his weight in gold every year,[9] history has consistently demonstrated that fatness is valued where wealth and plenty are hard to come by and fatness is a celebration of simply having enough to eat. It is no doubt true that these cultures value a bountiful harvest above mere human beauty but who can blame them when they are constantly faced with famine? When Gabrielle Palmer, nutritionist and author of *The Politics of Breastfeeding,*[10] was living in Mozambique, the African women were anxious and concerned about her as she is thin — ideal by Western standards. They kept pinching her to see if she had put on any weight and when she gained half a stone after a week eating peanuts, there was great rejoicing!

To contradict Arthur Marwick, it is *only* a society which values and actually has achieved wealth and status that can afford to idealise the thin body because there are no dangerously threatening associations with famine. In an affluent society, like that of Britain and America, restraint in eating becomes the symbol of social prestige. It can be interpreted as a symbolic statement that luxurious foods and physical languor are such everyday affairs that there is no need to overindulge in festival foods.[11] We have reached the stage of being able to play with food as an art form. We have invented *nouvelle cuisine*, and *cuisine minceur*, tiny portions of beautifully prepared food, arranged on the plate like a picture, often in the shapes of flowers, too pretty to eat and costing a great deal of money. We can toy with our food in this way because we have it in such abundance and we can strive to attain ultimate thinness because we do not need the primitive emergency reserves of fat to sustain us in times of shortage.

I was a child in the 1950s and I remember the post-war

rationing and the awareness that we had gone through a long period of shortages and deprivation. Food was valued and used with care. It could not be taken for granted. There was no room for faddiness. I remember my mother, who was a beautiful woman, wearing the full skirted dresses of that period, with the wide belts. At a size 12 she felt she was too thin and always wore padded bras to make her bust a good 36″. And we ate good, wholesome food.

Thirty-five years later we find the polarised situation where thin is so valued that a woman taking a size 36 bra writes a magazine article which begins: 'It is not easy in this world to have large breasts.'[12] The writer complains: 'Despite images in the media which represent an above average bust as desirable for women, the realities of owning such a commodity are painfully different.' Having decided to go and be measured properly for a correctly fitting bra, she finds–'to my relief' that she should wear a 36D. The assistant disappears, returning with 'a handful of donkey panniers'. The first one she tries fits and is beautifully comfortable. And she tells us what fun it is to do 'what no woman with big breasts ever thought she could — burn all the old bras'.

We are told that androgyny is out and that curves are back. Do not be deceived by this. If the writer of the above-mentioned article considers a 36D means she has big breasts, she is merely responding to the images fixed by the media as role models for modern woman; in 1992, top model Naomi Campbell was pronounced 'the perfect body' at 5′11″ and weighing 7½ stones (105lb).

THE MEDIA

Before the 1950s we did not recognize the immense power and influence which the media exerted on our culture. We had newspapers, wireless, and black and white television, which had not been around for very long. Then came more newspapers, magazines were born overnight, colour exploded onto our TV screens. Advertising became fiercely competitive and increasingly brilliant. We could not ignore the images that were being projected at us from all sides. And the Beautiful People, the wildly successful crop of thin sixties models set the trend. It is hard to resist media influence; it is intrusive, powerful, subliminal, fascinating. The world is indeed a stage now and we are in a position to see all the players. We are beguiled and bewitched by the kaleidoscope we see every day. We are presented with new goddesses — and they must not be fat. They must not even be normally healthy looking.

An example of this was the unrelenting newspaper and magazine obsession with the weight of both Diana, the Princess of Wales, and Sarah Ferguson, the Duchess of York. Diana was universally feted as 'beautiful' and 'a fairy-tale princess'; much was made of her clothes and her extreme slenderness. When there were rumours that she was anorexic, there was widespread concern. It later came to light that she was in fact, bulimic, and had been for very many years.[13]

The Duchess of York was invidiously compared with Diana at every opportunity. She was not fat by any definition, but she did put on weight when she was pregnant. Media idols — and these two young royal women were foremost in this category — are seen as gods and goddesses by our largely secular society, and they are expected to be beyond reproach, hardly human. To put on weight was a very ungoddess-like thing to do in the mind of the magazine and tabloid newspaper world and the message of retribution was clear — if goddesses fall from grace, they will be savagely attacked in print: 'From elegant to elephant in nine short months', and then 'From fat Fergie to svelte Sarah'. The tabloids dubbed her 'The Duchess of

Pork'.[14] And while Diana's suspected eating problem aroused only concern, Sarah's weight gain led to the most vitriolic attacks.

The visual media have brought us a long way from admiring the curving evidence of womanhood and fertility, even wishing us to deny the way Nature rounds our bodies in pregnancy itself. So conditioned is the modern figure-conscious woman that she often hates her pregnant shape and cannot distinguish the beautiful, swelling curve of the baby growing inside her from 'getting fat'. And so she is helped by magazines who recognize her distaste. *Vogue* shows her 'horseshoe neck tunics and empire line dresses which detract from the bulge' and recommends a designer who 'encourages reluctant mothers-to-be into black silk satin V-Shapes with lightly padded shoulders to detract from the bump'.

Every so often, the dictators of the fashion world pay lip-service to the return of the (slightly) larger figure. In a *Vogue* feature about the top models of 1988 the writer states that: 'None of these girls is remotely androgynous; unlike the skinny waifs of the early eighties they have proper figures — busts and hips that go in and out the way women are meant to.' Well at least that's an admission. And certainly the photographs of the models show them with fuller breasts than we have become accustomed to in fashion models. But as Jane Mulvagh, author of *The Vogue History of Twentieth Century Fashion*,[15] points out: 'aside from their pneumatic bosoms, many of these models are still impossibly thin — narrow-hipped and bird-limbed'. She goes on to say that a number of top models have confessed to having silicon breast implants: the new vogue for voluptuousness, she says, 'is an illusion. The contemporary ideal is still to be thin. To be thin — even unnaturally so — is to be relevant'. Jane Mulvagh goes on to say that well-designed clothes are for figures that rely on cigarettes and coffee to stave off hunger and stay at an 'ideal' yet artificially low weight. And this is far from being a 'model's disease' or an adolescent affliction, she says. 'Extreme thinness also infects middle-aged women who diet down to a size 8 in order to struggle into clothes designed for a teenaged body.'

Unliberated women are notoriously sheep-like when it comes to fashion. They collude with fashion designers and fashion journalists. 'Bad news this season for all those who have been growing their hair in order to be able to wear last year's longer styles,' I read, 'This year the styles are short.' Who assumes that women are going to have to cut their hair because fashion dictates this be so? It doesn't matter, because inevitably they do so, afraid of being anything less than trendy. And the fashion designer argues that it is not economical to accommodate the fluctuations of women's size and shape. He designs for a straight flat-chested girl because anyone with curves would only distort his intended silhouette.[16]

It disturbs me a great deal that the biggest 'normal' size — 14 — has now moved into the smallest 'large' size. In the early and mid-80s, the Big is Beautiful movement was proclaiming that 50 per cent of British women were a size 16 and over. Now that message has subtly changed to 60 per cent are size 14 and over. Size 14 means a 36″ bust and 38″ hips. Overweight? Fat? In 1960, Marilyn Monroe epitomised all that was enviable to women and desirable to men. The little black dress that she wore in 'Some Like it Hot' was displayed in an exhibition of costume. It was an outsize dress, a size 16. Five years later, in 1965, Twiggy arrived on the scene — 'six and a half stones (90lb) in weight . . . five foot six . . . dress size 6 . . . a thirty and a half inch bust and thirty-two inch hips'. In spite of car stickers which read Forget Oxfam: Feed Twiggy, thin was in to stay.[17]

The limits of acceptable normality in size are closing in. The media and fashion ideal is a cloned size 10 or even 8.

I asked a trendy friend in her early twenties about the sizes in boutiques. She — a size 10 — told me it was difficult to get anything above a twelve. And Evans, the chain for large British women, who used to be called — disgustingly — Evans Outsize until they had the decency to drop the tag several years ago, improved the image of their clothes when they improved their name and launched a new range of decent, middle of the road gear. At the same time they hung huge, fluorescent banners in all their stores — NOW AVAILABLE IN SIZE 14. This denotes several things, none of which is good news for fat women. If Evans are accommodating size 14 they have less room for clothes for us, women outside the normal size ranges. And although Evans claim to go up to a size 30, there are very few garments of that size available. They make no provision at all for the woman over size 30. According to Evans Head Office. 'Most of our customers would not identify with very large sizes — our average customer is a size 18.' I went along to my local branch to see what these average customers looked like. I know enough about large sizes to recognize that the shop was full of fat women, average size about 24 with the odd, relatively sylph-like size 18 drifting in or out. Evans had sent me a folder of their new season's fashions, photographed on a size 16-18 model. They did nothing for me because I could not identify with the clothes on women of that size. But I made straight for an assistant, about my size, wearing a gorgeous jewel-coloured dress that looked so good on her I could hardly bear to ask: Was it Evans? It was, they had it in stock and I bought two and love them, and wear them to feel good in.

The Big is Beautiful movement started in America with Carole Shaw who produced a fashion magazine, *Big and Beautiful Woman*. Nancy Roberts, Jewish-American, large, outrageous, warm and totally over the top took up the cause in Britain. Her message, like herself, was larger than life:

Why the hell *shouldn't* we be as valid as women, as sexual beings, as clothes wearers as any emaciated size 10? Why indeed, except that it takes courage, self-confidence, self-esteem and a willingness to raise two fingers to the self-satisfied 'normal' sizes. Nancy Roberts has been a trail-blazer. She presented a television series *Large as Life*. She instigated 'Big, Beautiful and Fit' dancing classes. She argued that there is no reason in the world that we should not wear a fire-engine red track suit if we want to and can find one. She wrote a book, partly autobiographical, partly inspirational. Like Nancy, the book is technicoloured, both in words and pictures.[18]

But — and I hesitate to sound like a damp rag both because I admire and am fond of Nancy and because I do believe she has done us a huge service — I have to remember the countrywomen I have talked to who would not feel right being as colourful and extrovert as Nancy. And the young women who have not enough sense of identity as yet to stray outside the one or two styles they feel safe in. I feel, too, that it needs to be said that it is so much easier to stand proud and confident as a fat woman if you are *tall*. Fat plus confidence equals Junoesque. It is a different thing if you are five foot three and weigh fifteen stones (210lb). Tall, fat women, confidently dressed with heads held high have a great deal of presence. The rest of us have an additional hurdle to overcome if we are short.

But the Big is Beautiful movement can teach us a lot. It can give us enough self-esteem to read the following with a mixture of disbelief and amusement, rather than listening to it, or heaven forbid, acting on it:

> Outsize or outcast? Clothes hunting for fruity figures is a formidable task . . . Many of us know that feeling in the changing room wondering why this dress just does not look as good as it did in the window . . . cuddly

shapes have their own rules. The idea is to aim for the silhouette of a long triangle [*God forbid*], beginning with wide boxy shoulders and skimming all the bulges to a point at your toes. To help achieve this think of these points:

THE DO'S
Introduce vertical lines wherever possible . . . and limit your colours, blending dark and bold shades. Now's the time to try out shoulder pads, a sharp and wider line at the shoulder will help clothes to hang smoothly away from your body, especially as you will now be wearing loose-fitting clothes which hide a multitude of sins [*there we go again*]. I'm sure you will see immediately how flattering this can be.

THE DON'TS
Horizontal lines are out, tucking is out, frills, gathers and tying in the middle are out. If you have to, then wide hip-slung belts or 20's style hip ties are a good compromise. Minimise clutter with less bulky fabrics and loose-cut woollies, don't mix patterns and textures, and no crossways stripes unless they are above the bust!

And finally?

Feel good about yourself; size is so unimportant.[19]

I immediately wanted to wear a cotton striped (horizontal of course) top with masses of pintucks, smocking, gathers and frills, a wide waist belt and a skirt of entirely different colour, pattern and texture, with as much clutter as I could find. I mentioned this to my friend Pamela. Then I noticed she wasn't laughing as I read the article to her. 'Well yes,' she said seriously to me. 'That's where so many fat people go wrong. Their clothes are too cluttered and they wear too many frills and flounces. They don't do anything for the figure.' My friend's unconscious endorsement of those who put fat people down by creating such rules for them had us both laughing. She can sit there, all fourteen stones (200lb) of her, being fattist with realizing it. And yet she accepts whatever criticisms of herself are thrown at her:

> I am a contradiction. I make all these remarks about fat people, but if they are made to me I accept them quite meekly. When I went to an orthopaedic specialist who said he wouldn't treat me until I lost weight, I went away agreeing with him.

> When women get together the talk often centers on weight and diets . . . There is no way I can describe on paper how this feels . . . The secret rage and humiliation of fat women could burn this country to the ground . . . Thin-identified women don't realise how political their fear of fat is . . . If the truth about fat and eating were known, thin women would only be able to consider themselves lucky, not especially deserving, and the system of belief in individual struggle and individual achievement . . . would be broken down.
>
> Vivian Mayer (Aldebaran), Feminist and Fat Activist, quoted in a speech by Dr Wayne Wooley 2 September 1979 at the NAAFA Convention in Arlington, Virginia

Where fashion is concerned my friend feels that the fat woman has an obligation to others. She believes she has already offended their eye by her size, so she should seek to compensate for this by making the best of herself in the areas of hair, make-up, etc. Pamela believes that we, as fat women, do not have the right to look just as we want to, in the way our thin sisters do. She herself, while provoking many a laugh at her revelations of unconscious fat prejudice, nevertheless imposes on herself those standards of appearance she would like to see imposed on other fat women. Whichever way you look at the issue of fat it comes back to the same root — that of sinning. Pamela, like so many, believes we must do penance by pleasing society in those areas we can change — clothes, face, hair — and not cause further offence by transgressing the fat fashion rules.

Insecurities amongst fat women are random and surprising. Pamela does not consciously mind about being fat, whereas I who do mind would not consider wearing make-up, because I do not like it. I don't feel I have to present a good face just to please others. Lee, who is a feminist and who would like the freedom to dispense with make-up also feels she must wear it, though it does not form part of her overall image. It is another apologetic placatory advance to society, a tiny proof that she is doing something to conform even while she is failing in the main area of size and shape. This is what society does to us and we respond to its bullying demands in different ways.

Five feet two and size 18 — I draw the line at that.

Designer Bruce Oldfield

One American designer is renowned for declaring that if a woman doesn't have enough self-respect to starve herself into a size 12, he for one doesn't want the out-of-control slob wearing his clothes.

The Times 20 April 1992

I once sat through a miserable lunch with the fashion editor of a glossy magazine during which she told me in great detail how I could improve myself, and in fact wanted me to become a model for a magazine 'make-over', those awful before and after beauty sessions where the pictures before always look so much more attractive to me than the artificial 'after' results. Remembering that lunch gives me a milestone on the road to improving my self-esteem: it may not be high as yet, but were that same occasion to occur now I would have the courage to tell the woman that I am happy with my hair and face the way it is, that I don't want a perm or contact lenses or make-up. Pamela, hypothetically faced with the same situation would feel obliged to comply; being fat has stripped her of her own visual identity.

In these subtle ways and a million others we are cajoled by the mainstream of society to conform where we can, even while we commit one major sin. I am glad that I can laugh at articles which talk about the Do's and Don'ts of fashion rules for 'fatties', and I think the Big is Beautiful movement is responsible for a great deal of that. Fat women find it all too easy to fall into the trap of believing that they have fewer rights than their slim sisters whom they think of as being free to get up, pull on a pair of jeans, run a comb through unstyled hair and go out, unmade-up and unapologetic.

In many ways what I have said about the liberating influence of the Big is Beautiful movement is rather different, I think, from the message the movement itself intended to convey. It is common for fat women to have such a low self-esteem that they do not consider that it is worth beautifying something that is basically 'faulty' or deformed; the thinking is something on the opposite lines of gilding the lily. So because they are fat, and perhaps cannot wear the clothes they would like to, they do not consider it worth having the hair style they would like or paying attention to beauty care. And so Big is Beautiful says: 'Love your size, pamper your body, decorate it, show it off, if you've got it, flaunt it — you have as much right as any woman born to make the best of yourself, to enhance your assets'. And that message is *right*. Fat women are liable to be labouring either side of the delusion: that they are not worth 'beautifying' or that they *have* to make an attempt rather than compound their felony.

My uneasiness about the Big is Beautiful movement is that I think it smacks of positive discrimination and denies fat people their true identities. I do not feel it is helpful to any oppressed minority who just wants to take its place alongside the rest of the world. It has to do with belonging and equality. To say that Big or Black or Jewish or older women are beautiful or 'better than' is to remove that section of society, to cordon it off in effect into its own enclave, to remove it from prejudice and condemnation but to replace it just as firmly outside the fence of heterogeneity, but in a different place. I do not believe Big is Beautiful. I believe it is normal and therefore worthy of the same unexceptional treatment as those whom society already considers normal. I would like to see fat people accorded a validity which has nothing to do with their size or their looks. That, the way I see it, is true equality.

Until 1986 there was no women's publication in Britain that catered for the fashion, psychology and general needs of 'the larger lady'. Women's magazines carried the occasional article about large-size clothes but there were no positive role models for fat women. In 1984 Eleanor Graham, a public relations consultant, arranged a British tour for Carole Shaw, editor of the American *Big and Beautiful Woman*. Wherever Carole Shaw appeared with her message that fat women could survive and bloom in a world obsessed with thinness, hundreds of letters poured into the television and radio stations, newspapers and magazines where she had left her mark. It was obvious that over half the women in Britain wanted something for themselves, the size 16 pluses.

Eleanor Graham realized that here was a huge and unfilled gap in the British media market and she set about filling it. To her astonishment, in spite of the response to Carole Shaw, no British publishing house was interested in launching a similar magazine. Eleanor, herself a large woman with integrity, anger and enormous determination on her side, took out a massive overdraft and launched her own magazine *Extra Special*. Her first discovery was that there were no large models so, undaunted, she advertised for 'real people' and held auditions for the amateurs who turned up.

The magazine was a joy for fat women — it contained clothes modelled on real women with fat bodies and wide, un-model like smiles. The features were uncompromising: 'Be large, be healthy: it just isn't true that larger means less fit' and 'How dieting can make you fat'. There was an agony aunt for fat women's emotional problems and a practising psychotherapist, herself a fat woman. Eleanor Graham's editorial message was clear:

> To weigh more than nine stones risks a 'Fatty' label: the larger woman has been made to feel guilty and inferior. The fashion press ignores her. The multi-million pound slimming industry preys upon her. She is the butt of cheap sit-com jokes. We think this is absurd. It insults half the healthy normal women in the land. It is dangerous because it can cause them needless stress and pressurises them into unnecessary and useless dieting.

There was more in the same vein, and Eleanor concluded:

> If you want help in dieting, do not come to us, try your doctor. We will take weight off where it really matters

— off your mind. We are here to help you lead the full life that you are entitled to live without worry, pretence or apology.

After the first issue, the letters poured in. The following one sums up the messages contained in all of them:

I was so overjoyed by my first copy of marvellous *Extra Special* that I sat down and wept. You have made sense out of my muddled idea that nobody else in the world felt as I did. I felt that being large meant I was gross, ugly and an outsider. *Extra Special* has brought sanity and fresh air into my life. Thank you for giving me back my self-respect.

Extra Special sold well, though Eleanor could only afford to bring it out bi-monthly. Reader response continued to be excited, grateful, confident, positive. Then in 1988 Robert Maxwell made Eleanor Graham an offer for the magazine. She did not want to sell because she feared that its message and its image would change, but she also knew that Maxwell was capable of bringing out his own magazine in competition and as a private entrepreneur she could not have weathered that. So she sold, retaining a position as PR consultant. The magazine moved into the Maxwell empire, though he was touchy about advance publicity; he did not like the idea of being photographed with a fat woman. The title was retained but the first issue was glossier, slicker and reflected some of Eleanor's fears. It disguised frank fatness with unreal, glamorous images. Then, without warning, Maxwell axed it. There was no second issue, no explanation. The editorial staff found themselves unemployed. There was nowhere for disappointed readers to write to, readers who had been waiting in anticipation for issue no. 2.

And the gap in the market yawned wide again. Was it political? Is it possible that a magazine for and about frankly fat women, which was triumphantly gaining success and status, was too offensive to be allowed to continue in a media world which abhors fatness?

There is no doubt about the media's fear of fatness. Since the original launch of *Extra Special* there has been a spate of newspaper articles paying tribute to 'Big is Beautiful'. But more often than not this is no more than tokenism. A newspaper fashion feature called 'As Large As Life'[20] waxed excited about French model Valerie Rousseaux. 'Big is being taken seriously in the thinnest fashion circles', this article states and goes on to say that Valerie Rousseaux turned up for a photo session wearing a skirt that hovered six inches above her shapely knees. And while that in itself would not be enough to excite comment the fact is that Valerie is a size 18, and such is received opinion about what big girls ought to wear that she set up 'something of a rumpus in her wake'. Not it seems because she was a fat woman wearing a short skirt, but because she looked 'curvaceously fabulous, enough to make men boggle and women envious'. The sight of her, the journalist claims, is enough to demolish fashion's discriminatory arguments against large sizes at a single glance. While admitting that Valerie Rousseaux is a special case, a model and a 'peachy-skinned' nineteen year old, the journalist contends that her very presence on the modelling scene should be proof for the huge number of ordinary big women that their sentence as fashion outcasts is — gradually — coming to an end.

I don't believe a word of this. For a start, Mlle Rousseaux has the huge eyes and fine features of any fashion model. She is tall, her limbs are slim and elegant. I cannot imagine that any doctor would suggest she lose weight. She is simply not as unnaturally, anorexically thin as most fashion models. I cannot imagine how the 'ordinary big women' would be able to identify with her. We, as fat women, do not have the experience of being 'enough to make men boggle and women envious'. If it were so, I should not have any reason to write this book or you to read it.

About once a year a British newspaper, usually one of the tabloids, will run a feature on 'large-size models', each time proclaiming this as a new fashion trend. Apparently we now have 'the first up-market outsize model agency in the country' which is planning to use girls who are 'curvy, womanly and voluptuous'. According to the article which reports on this, the new agency 'may be a positive step forward in people's conception of fat women'.[21]

While these women may be larger than the traditional models (who, incidentally, are usually underweight for their height even by the standards of the unrealistic Metropolitan Life Insurance charts) they are by no means fat — they are tall, as models always are, and size 14–18.

I am disturbed by this. By stating that the use of average as opposed to underweight models may be a step forward in popular conception of what defines a fat woman, this confirms the view that many women hold as gospel: that to be size 14 or 16 is to be fat. And if women of that size define themselves as fat, there has to be a line drawn — between them and us, as it were. That line is found in the statement made by one agency owner who has big and beautiful models, 'none of whom could ever be insultingly described as obese'.[22] This is why we cannot identify with these women as role models. Their size–weight–height ratio means that they are not stigmatised or derided.

Nowhere in the modelling business do we find the beautiful large, fat and super-sized women that *Extra Special* used to feature, and which *Radiance* and *Pretty Big* do. Even these token 'large-size' models will never replace the slim ones, says the writer of the article, 'no matter how stunning the face . . . with ingrained images of thinness being equal to beauty in the minds of most'.

Magazines are even worse than newspapers. Even *Country Living*, which ran a patronising and incongruous feature: 'Accentuate the Positive. If you're big, shout about it.' Encouraging, don't you agree? The feature goes into the lives of women who are large, like a fashion student who has longed to fit into trendy clothes and look like a model, but believes that dream is not worth starving and suffering for. The real problem is clothes for her size, she says, as does the journalist who says that it is really important to be the person you are. Another interviewee does not believe in slimming rules for large women and wears bright colours because she wants to be seen. Another has red hair which she wears long and bushy to detract from her large bottom. She doesn't diet a lot because you can really get to dislike your body if you do that and she feels that women should not be made to feel they must conform to a single image. There follows advice for large women on giving themselves permission to look wonderful by using colour boldly, and on looking after their bodies, keeping them healthy and in good condition.

Why am I so angry at this particular feature? Because the women interviewed are all a size 14 and absolutely stunning. They are not large. They are just not anorexic.

The worst offender was *Elle* magazine, which was using models so impossibly thin and tall that it was rumoured that some sneaky stretching of the photographs had taken place, and *Cosmopolitan*, both sides of the Atlantic. Helen Gurley Brown, who launched *Cosmopolitan* in America, is widely held to abhor fat; to be 'fatphobic'. An American television documentary on weight issues interviewed Brown and hypothesised that more than any other individual in America she might deserve 'credit' for the epidemic of eating disorders amongst young American women.[23] In what can only be described as a less-than-token attempt to acknowledge that the tide might be turning, *Cosmopolitan* reported on the demonstrations against dieting in which American women burned diet books and smashed scales. 'But do they feel better for it?', the reporter asks patronisingly, 'Are they now happily stuffing cream cakes without a care?' (the usual gluttonous assumptions before the article has got under way). It continues: 'It would be wonderful to say that size doesn't matter — personality and intelligence are far more important.' Aren't they? Apparently not. 'It's a fact that today, as at any time in history, there exists a physical ideal.' But *Cosmopolitan* condescendingly offers us hope: 'Cindy Crawford (top model) has even revealed that there are days, while doing fashion photography, when she has to hold her stomach in . . .'. And *Cosmo*'s large models are 'around 5'10" with a 36" bust'. Cindy Crawford says 'We focus on our ugliness', so *Cosmo* urges us, 'Okay, maybe you are a size 16, but you might have thick, glossy hair and slender calves, so you should make the most of them.'[24]

I'd like to say just one thing to *Cosmopolitan* and other similar glossy women's magazines. Maybe we are a size 16, or 18, or 30, or 40. And maybe we look absolutely beautiful. Without even having to search for 'compensating features', like glossy hair. Maybe we can make the most of *ourselves* just as we are.

Fortunately we have *YES* and *Pretty Big* magazines, relatively new on the scene and fighting for us, and the American *Radiance* which is positive, warm and militant in its fight against all forms of fattism. These magazines feature glorious clothes in large sizes.

TELEVISION, FILM AND NOVELS

Our view of the world is, like it or not, largely formed and influenced by the visual media, particularly television which is for most people an essential part of home life. Whether we realize it or not, it is pervasive and to some extent invasive. Television, like most women's magazines, is an *intimate* medium; it communicates directly to us, right into our homes; it becomes part of the fabric of our lives and increasingly, it invites us to take part in the life on screen. Since the advent of daytime television, the magazine programmes and chat shows ask us the viewers to communicate as well, to write or phone, and now to participate in live phone-ins. One minute we could be watching a programme; the next, we could be part of it, airing our opinions and feelings, helping shape the direction of that particular show or segment.

This ever-increasing two-way communication has the effect of 'dissolving' the screen, the barrier between 'them' and 'us'. With its high output of dramas, serials, series and soap operas, television portrays a microcosm of the world with which the viewer identifies. The art of television is an attempt to imitate life; this is particularly so in seriously realistic dramas. And because television is such an influential medium, people unconsciously aspire to be like the characters portrayed, whether real or fictitious. And so life imitates art and the cycle continues.

The fat woman watching television will notice, consciously or unconsciously, that she is absent from this portrayal of life. The more informal television becomes, and the more intimately it reaches into our lives, the more invisible grows the fat woman. There are no fat newsreaders — though they are not necessarily glamorous, or young, or white. There are no fat presenters, even though they may seem homely and approachable and mention their own problems in a way that suggests they are just ordinary women like the rest of us. The reporter, speaking live out in the open somewhere, hair blowing wildly in the wind, is not glamorous. But she is thin. We watch plays, films, soaps and see wives, mothers, lovers, career women, girlfriends. Where are we represented? Do we really exist?

The answer is yes, we have been given a place on television, but only in one of three clearly defined roles. We can be shown in a low-status job — the two most popular soap operas in Britain have both had fat barmaids — Pam St. Clement in BBC's *EastEnders*, and Betty Turpin in *Coronation Street* on ITV. Alternatively, we can be seen in our compensating personality roles — the Earth Mother and the Joker, translated for television to the Agony Aunt who advises viewers on their problems, and the comedienne. On British television, Claire Rayner is a familiar figure in the former part, popping up all over the place. And Denise Robertson does the job for *This Morning*, ITV's daytime magazine programme.

There are numerous comediennes on television. Some like Grotbags, the Green Witch on children's television are made to look hideous or ridiculous. Some, like Bella Emberg who appears with Russ Abbott, make a point of drawing self-deprecating attention to their size by the use of fat jokes. And some are very funny and very clever, like Dawn French and Jo Brand (who once answered the question 'Would you take a magic pill to make you thin?' with a laconic 'No. I'd rather have a cake.')

Take just one of these examples, Dawn French, one of the most popular women on British television. Her material is of a high standard, she has terrific reviews, journalists always want to write about her — she is a high profile and much-respected celebrity. Her size is acknowledged but not ridiculed (though it is worth pointing out here that Dawn French is not very fat). Dawn is more of a comic actress than a comedienne and the material she writes and performs herself does not focus on her size. The parts she writes are for a woman, not a fat woman. Yet she is sent endless scripts for consideration, all with parts for a fat woman. She cannot understand why fat actresses are excluded from all 'normal' female roles. She longs to play Kate in Shakespeare's *The Taming of The Shrew*, but it is considered outside her 'type'. Yet no-one *knows* that Kate was thin.

Annette Badland, another talented British actress has faced the same stereotyping and discrimination. She played a moronic maid in a television adaptation of an Agatha Christie thriller (the book does not suggest that the maid was fat, merely dim); in a bad sit-com about a wives group, she represented the slow and stupid member; and she was thoroughly miscast in purple crimplene in the TV dramatisation of Ian McEwan's powerfully black story *The Last Day of Summer*. Set in the 1960s in a hippy commune, the play observes the friendship which develops between the two people who don't belong — a ten-year-old boy, and Annette's fat character. In the filming, Annette was made to exaggerate being fat — she is seen puffing and panting as she walks and climbs stairs — she normally has no trouble with these activities. Camera angles are carefully aimed to show incongruous close-ups of solid lumps of flesh and of the sweat pouring from her. It is a gross parody of a fat woman. In the end, she falls out of a boat — it is not quite clear how, or why — and dies an ignominious death. Justice for the sinner, perhaps? Annette has been cast as the fat woman in a *radio* play, as though there are 'fat' voices, and she failed the audition for a play *reading* she was particularly keen to do because the author said her character would not have been fat.

'Who listens to fat women?'

> Character in 'Fat Chance', an episode of *Inspector Morse*. ITV
> Channel 4, 8 September 1993

In *Bergerac*, the long-running detective series set on the Channel Island of Jersey, Annette played the filing clerk in the police office. In the third series a rare and enlightened producer recognized her talent and saw it was being wasted. He gave her character more prominence, her part developed and grew, and she was even allowed to fall in love. In the fourth series the producer was replaced and this one wanted Annette tucked back among the filing cabinets where he thought she belonged. She resigned from *Bergerac* on principle, a courageous decision in a precarious profession made more so by the limitations imposed upon her because of her size.

Any proof needed that the stereotyped media ideal is forced upon women only can be found in the complete inequality of male and female roles. In straight drama, as opposed to character acting or comedy, fat men can be seen in normal situations, playing normal people — mirroring life, in fact. In the last-ever series of the immensely popular *Inspector Morse*, which was shown on British television in January 1993, there was one episode with three very fat men in serious, authoritative parts: James Grout had been Morse's Chief Superintendent throughout; Richard Griffiths played an eminent Oxford clergyman who was also an academic with specialist knowledge; and the pathologist, though he appeared in only one scene, was also fat. When I say fat, with regard to these three men, I do not mean portly, or well-built. All three were very fat, but their size neither detracted from nor added to their characters. I am sure the only reason I noticed them was because I am aware of these things; my husband, when I asked him, had not noticed their size. He would have done, however, if the same parts had been taken by fat women, not because it would have been incongruous in itself, but because it is unprecedented. Certainly three fat women in one programme, all playing serious and respected characters, would have been a television phenomenon.

It will not happen overnight, but there are cracks

appearing, making way for more positive fat role-models. Roseanne Barr has been immensely popular both sides of the Atlantic, and though she too is playing for laughs, she has a real-life part — she is a wife and mother and friend who succeeds and fails in the daily round and the common task no more and no less than the media's definition of the 'normal' woman. It is America which is leading the field in this revolution — and it is coming from successful American actresses who are tired of the equation of slimness with normality and success. In a startling episode of the popular drama series, 'LA Law', actress Susan Peretz successfully sued her former employer for dismissing her because of her weight. In an interview with *Radiance* magazine, Peretz said she had spent 20 years being typecast in character roles but that she does feel that attitudes are changing slowly.[26]

Another American series, *Designing Women*, also ran a much-publicised episode addressing fat oppression. This was the actress Delta Burke's response to real life attacks on the weight she gained during the series. American tabloids went to town, knocking her self-esteem and saying her weight gain had landed her in marriage trouble. The malice directed at the actress came from all sides; some radio stations broadcast a jingle — 'Delta Dawn, how many pounds have you put on'. With her producer, Linda Bloodworth-Thomason, Delta Burke tackled the issue in an episode set at a high-school reunion. Her character, Suzanne Sugarbaker, is the target of mocking and unpleasant remarks from former classmates and then voted 'the most changed' of the group. In a scene which brought a standing ovation from the studio audience, Suzanne Sugarbaker speaks out for Delta Burke — and for all of us: 'Drugs, alcohol . . . whatever your problems, people are sympathetic. Unless you're fat. Then you're supposed to be ashamed . . . I don't want to feel like I have to be thin in order to be loved and admired.' The episode unleashed a deluge of emotional viewer response from fat women who for once saw their plight represented in that most highlighted arena — the television series.

The hit song, 'Gonna Make You Sweat' by the group C&C Music Factory, has some 'awesome' female vocals on it, sung by Martha Wash, who is fat. But her name does not appear on the album cover, and she does not tour with the group. When this song is performed in concert, Martha Wash's vocals are mimed by Zelma Davis, a thin woman. Ms Davis also appears in the group's video, lip-synching Martha Wash's vocals. Freedom Williams, the group's male lead singer, was asked on television to give the reasons for replacing Martha Wash on the video and in stage appearances. He replied: 'She sings very well, but all the men in the audience, me included, would much rather watch Zelma's body than Martha's.'

NAAFA Newsletter, May 1991

Each time an actress departs from the glamorous stereotype in which she has been cast, we are a step further towards becoming visible. Two extremes come to mind: in the film *Death Becomes Her*, Goldie Hawn wore a fat-suit because her character put on a great deal of weight. When she first stepped into the suit, Ms Hawn is reported to have panicked, though I am not clear why, and 'for a moment it looked as though the $200,000 suit might have to be scrapped'.[27] This does not exactly help our cause. On the other hand, Sharon Gless, the slim and glamorous half of *Cagney and Lacey*, deliberately gained about three stones (40lb) for her role as the bingeing, crazy, book-fanatic in Stephen King's play *Misery* which opened in London in

January 1993. Ms Gless was unconcerned about her weight gain; it was necessary for the part and she knew she would lose it in time. The person who *did* mind was her husband, Barney Rosenzweig. He did not like it at all. Though even with 40 extra pounds, Sharon Gless was by no stretch of the imagination fat.

Britain has one glorious fat heroine on screen — Pam Ferris, playing Ma Larkin in H.E. Bates's *The Darling Buds of May*. This has been one of the biggest successes on British television, evoking, as it does, a nostalgic way of life, where the pace was slow and family relationships meant everything, and food was both an art form and one of life's greatest pleasures. Pam Ferris herself has spoken out publicly on behalf of the maligned 'overweight', challenging the assumptions of thinness being good. She is anti-diet, and very opposed to any kind of persecution or persuasion of fat people. Her creed is 'live and let live'.

Outside television drama we *do* have some wonderful role models. In Britain, the tap-dancing group, the Roly Polys, led by Mo Moreland, is truly astonishing. Mo gives the lie to all the myths about being fat and unhealthy. She is *very* fat and she is short, well under 5 feet. And she is not young — she is well into her 60s. But she and the other Roly Polys, who are also fat, go through tap-dancing routines which would have the majority of 'normal'weight people lying on the floor gasping for breath. They also have a punishing touring schedule, home and abroad.

America has an inspirational group of performers, The Fat Lip Readers Theater Group. The 13 or so members vary in age, colour, sexual preference, class and profession. Some are able-bodied, others disabled. The two things they have in common is that they are fat and they are talented. A performance consists of singing, dancing and acting. They write their own material and their skits are about what it is like to be a fat woman in America. They are clever and very funny and their audiences laugh, identify and sometimes weep. In some ways they resemble Britain's Spare Tyre Theatre Company, except that Fat Lip women are *fat!* I would love an opportunity to perform with them. It brings home the fact that amateur theatre groups would not know what to do with a fat woman if they didn't just happen to have a typecast character part for her!

Maria Callas, the great opera singer, lost 62 lb using the tapeworm cure. This entailed swallowing a tablet containing an embryonic tapeworm, which when grown to fullsize would eat the food eaten by its human host. In the 1920s, three out of five dieters were using tapeworms, despite warnings issued by the American Medical Association. Not surprisingly, the tapeworms caused chronic inflammation of the stomach and malnutrition. Callas's biographer, Michael Scott, founder of the London Opera Society, argues that the singer was only any good vocally when she was fat and says that it is not an accident that Pavarotti is stout — the voice, to a large extent, is suited to the figure. The physical body supports the voice. 'She'd built up a voice to suit her size and then she took it all away' says Scott.

Tyranny of Beauty, Arline and John Liggett (Gollancz Books, 1982), and
Fat Power, Louderback (NY Hawthorn, 1970).

A couple of years ago I turned on the radio and heard the most wonderful voice — rich, haunting, compelling and unlike any other I had heard. It was Canadian Rita MacNeil singing her hit song *Working Man* and I wanted to hear more of that voice. I discovered that she was Canada's top female singer and that she was very fat. She too is an inspiration, not because of her voice itself, but because she has not let her size stop her from using that voice, standing on a concert platform alone and carrying on, despite reviewers' constant references to her size. It has been all the more difficult for her because she is shy and naturally reserved, but if she hadn't pushed through that and all the prejudice against being fat and over 40, we would have been deprived of something very special.

> This film is about what society does to women by telling them from earliest childhood that their whole future happiness, their potential to find contentment and love, has to do with how many inches there are around their hips.
>
> Henry Jaglom, on his film, *Eating* (*Sunday Express*, 7 July 1991)

These women show that it can be done against all the odds.

Is film any better? I think there are brave attempts on the part of film-makers in progress, helped by the emergence of a truly beautiful and very fat film actress, Marianne Sagebrecht. Her first big part in *Sugarbaby* looked superficially hopeful. She played a normal woman who had a normal relationship. But in the end the film conformed to expected media stereotype; she may have got her man but she lost him. Her next film was excitingly different. *Bagdad Cafe* came to England in 1989 and was received with loud praise for the sensitive handling of the friendship between two women, and for the sheer beauty of Sagebrecht herself and her acting. No marginalisation there, but a *real* triumph.

Search hard enough and you can even find the occasional surprise in fiction. One of the most ritzy, glitzy books of 1989 was *Kiss and Tell*.[28] A story of scandal and sexual politics where journalists climb to the top of their profession bed by bed. One of the main characters is Ruth, fashion editor, the best in the business, sought after by rival newspapers. Brilliant at her job, with masses of friends, lovers and finally a husband and baby, Ruth is fat, not large or plump, but really fat. And she gets the best of everything. Struck down by illness she loses all the weight she has, but when she recovers she puts it all back on and enjoys it. I wish I knew if she is based on anyone. The only large fashion editor I ever knew got the sack for it though she was only size 16.

Then there was Susan Sussman's *The Dieter* which is about friendship, and loss, about families and husbands and lovers, and about food, the way we use it and the tyranny of slimming clubs and diet plans. And Sherry Ashworth's triumphant first novel, *A Matter of Fat*, published first by a local co-operative then bought for the mass market by Penguin because it is so good. It is the story of the women who attend a slimming club (a marvellous take-off of Weight Watchers) and of the club's leader and her ambitions. The moral of this hugely moving and entertaining novel is that diets don't work and being thin is not what life is about.

It is essential that the fat woman's place in society be represented in the media so that she sees herself existing in the roles allotted to so-called 'normal' women. This is more important now than it has ever been, because fat women are the only group still barred from a society ostensibly committed to equal opportunities.

The media is blamed for holding up an impossible ideal of thinness, causing the ever-widening anorexia epidemic. The irony here is that the anorexic's real aim is to have no body at all. No weight is ever low enough for her; at some deep level she wants to disappear, to be invisible, to be a creature of mind and spirit without matter. Yet she is saved from this annihilation by a cloak of attention, concern and fascination. She will become part of 20th-century romantic mythology, just as the anorexic saints and fasting girls of the past have done. The fat woman, though, whose body is objectively perceived as unacceptable, occupies only an empty space. Without this life-affirming feedback, her psyche, if not her body, is in danger of disappearing. To see oneself *absent*, outside the boundaries of human life causes a feeling of unreality, and of annihilation. It endangers the soul.

ADVERTISING

The problem with media images is that everyone is so dependent on advertising. And that really is the bottom line because that is where the real fat hatred is. I telephoned Mediatypes, a London agency specialising in jobs in advertising and public relations. I spoke to a genuinely helpful woman who assured me that she could get me a good job with my qualifications and experience. I must be honest with you, I told her. I am very fat. Will that make a difference? She told me that it made her very angry but that yes, it would debar me from any sort of job like that. The briefs were very specific, she said, as to the sort of appearance required in women in that profession. They really did want the tall, slim blonde stereotypes even though half the female consumers are size 16 plus.

Why? In an article in *Extra Special* in October 1988, Dan Donohue, Vice Chairman of McCormick Publicity attempted to explain the advertising rationale. Advertisers, he said, are very concerned with associating their products with people who are aspirational. The idea is not to be realistic (he said it), depicting an accurate picture, warts and all, but to create a glossy, fantasy world where everything is brighter and more beautiful. The emphasis, he said, is strongly on youth, fashion and fitness. Large women just are not symbolic of any of these qualities in the public consciousness.

That sounds to me like an example of making the tail wag the dog. The public consciousness takes its cue from advertising and media images, not the other way round. A senior planner at another agency confirmed this, saying that in aspirational advertisements only the 'sublimely beautiful' will do, and in 'average' advertisements an 'ordinarily pretty, non-head-turning actress is selected'. And 'average' in most creative and casting directors' minds is a size 8/10 so that is what they go for: 'When so many people are waging a constant war with their weight, no-one wants to run the risk of implying that using a particular product might result in a bulging waistline.' Fat, bad and dangerous to know, that's what we are, obviously. In Spain they have a better sense of proportion. The Jane Fonda look has not caught on at all there. Mercedes Sanchez, a copywriter based in Salamanca explained:

> Because our attitude to weight is very much more relaxed, our scripts very often call for shapely ladies to contribute their very special brand of sensuality. Food is part and parcel of hospitality, harmony, love and seduction. Viewers respond to a woman who looks as if she is capable of profound emotion.

In the February 1989 issue, *Options* magazine put three top advertising agencies to the test. Could they produce images concerned with concepts firmly rooted in reality? In other words, what could they come up with when asked to produce an advertisement promoting a positive image of fat? The results showed, in my opinion, a complete inability to step into the real world, a certain amount of prejudice against fat and a total lack of creativity.

The first, from Abbott, Mead Vickers/SMS Ltd featured a simple line drawing of a slim fountain pen with a pair of feet and arms and a female head. The main caption read:

'Nobody ever penned a poem to a girl built like a pen' and a smaller line underneath: 'Curves are in, weight is great.' The irony about this one is the metaphor chosen. The term 'pencil-slim' is totally complimentary and usually bestowed with a hint of envy.

The second advertisement took one of the standard *negative* images of fat — a pig — and captioned it: 'When did you last see an unhappy pig?' The copy was full of unconvincing 'advantages' of being fat, and ended with the (again negative) line: 'Remember, it's easy to scoff' (meaning to eat — like a pig, I presume). This example of unconscious prejudice came from the Thatcher image-makers, Saatchi and Saatchi. I find it totally unconvincing, like the leaderene herself.

The last advertisement featured a plumpish naked woman throwing open a pair of louvred doors, and says simply: 'Being more of a woman doesn't make you less of a person' — and underneath: 'Health education.' This came from WCRS Matthews, Marcantio Ltd.

It was an interesting and original exercise by *Options* magazine and I do wonder how much these awful images of fat resulted from lack of imagination on the part of their creators and how much from fear of creating a beautiful, positive image which just might make people think differently.

What else, though, can you expect from a profession that 'sacked' Winnie the Pooh, the Gales Honey emblem and mascot? The pronouncement on Pooh was that he looked 'fat, self-indulgent and unfit'.[29] They want honey to be seen as a natural, fitness-inspiring food and seem to think that if we see Pooh eating their honey we will not buy it for fear that we shall also become fat. Would consumers really respond to the Pooh Bear image in the way Gales feared they would? If so, there lies as much madness and fat-phobia in the general public as in the advertising profession.

6

Your loss is their gain: diets and the dieting industry

Diane is 41, and works several hours a week as a 'daily' in the village where she was born and still lives. She is a good-looking woman, tall, rosy-cheeked and very large indeed. She is happily married and has one daughter:

I've always been big — all the women in my family are. Being fat doesn't worry me at all — not for myself, that is. And Jim likes me the way I am — I think a lot of men like big women, really. He likes something to get hold of! We both like our food and I love cooking. I hated the time after I left school and was working. I just wanted to settle down and have a home of my own with a husband and children. I'm not very ambitious, but I'm not clever, so why should I be? People these days don't accept that you can be content being a housewife and looking after a family. Perhaps they're all from London where women have careers and families. They ought to take a look at ordinary country people. I like pottering about at home and earning a bit of extra money cleaning. I get plenty of exercise walking to work — I don't drive and the lady I clean for lives two miles away, just outside the village, *and* it's uphill!

If it was up to me and Jim I would never worry about being big, but it's other people, isn't it? They make me feel guilty about being fat, as though I've done something very wrong. It's enough to drive you to eating. I've tried to diet so many times. The money I've wasted on different ways of losing weight — trying to please other people! Is it really up to us to get thin for them, or should society change its attitude towards us?

When Kate Moss arrived on the scene last year (1992), with her flat chest, bandy legs, pale face and large sunken eyes, the size 8 coathanger was back in business . . . Cindy Crawford, slim by anyone's standards, was pronounced fat, while Rachel Hunter, a small size 12 was used to model outsize clothes. Women everywhere were in a mad panic, and models themselves realised that to stay in business they had to lose pounds fast . . . Yasmin Le Bon . . . has been known to faint with hunger at photo shoots. Elle McPherson, better known as The Body, used to smoke 60 cigarettes a day . . . others resort to drugs such as speed, and in New York and Milan, cocaine use is reported as widespread among models to promote weight loss . . . Says Linda Hartley, a model in the 1980s with Bookings agency in London: 'I remember being on a job in Tokyo with some other models. We went out for a meal and every single girl went to the bathroom afterwards and threw up. That's common.'

Sunday Times (London), 9 May 1993

Diane's unhappiness about the pressure put on her from outside has caused her to develop an unbalanced eating pattern, with yo-yo dieting and bouts of compulsive eating. Consequently her relationship with food is a struggle between her natural enjoyment of cooking — and eating a large amount of good food — and her feelings of 'oughts' and 'shoulds' which now surround her eating. Because she has become conditioned to being unable to be relaxed about eating, food looms large in her life and most of the time she worries about it.

She would have been doing so to the same extent had she lived 100 years ago. Dieting really took off in the middle of the 19th century, both in Britain and the United States. Graham crackers were one of the first American diet foods, patented by a clergyman, the Reverend Sylvester Graham, who railed against gluttony. Over in Britain, a well-known London undertaker, William Banting, was fretting about his own increasing girth and his deafness. The latter was diagnosed as a direct result of the former, 'adipose matter in the throat pressing upon the Eustachian tubes'. Banting went on a regime which excluded farinaceous and saccharine foods — in other words, carbohydrates. He lost weight, rejoiced and wrote *Letter on Corpulence* which sold over 58,000 copies. Thus began the dieter's preoccupation with avoiding starchy foods, which persisted until the 1980s. So popular was Banting's diet that 'banting' entered the language on both sides of the Atlantic as a verb. There are people alive today who can remember 'banting' being talked about, and practised by their mothers and their friends.

Anti-fat remedies abounded, particularly in the United States. Some were intended to attack the offending flesh *in situ*. There was Every Woman's Flesh Reducer, for instance, a bath powder with citric acid, Epsom salts, camphor, soda and alum. Or Absorbit Reducing Paste with oxbile, beeswax and lard, and Fatoff, 90 per cent water and 10 per cent soap. There were obesity powders, laxatives and enemas, and faradic treatment (electric currents applied to the body, including *inside* the uterus), but nothing worked. 'I have tried everything you ever tried,' bewailed one woman in 1914. 'I went through exercises, rolled on the floor, cut down my food, gave up sweets, fats and starches, wore elastic clothing, tried electricity, massage, osteopathy, vibration, hot and vapor baths, swallowed pellets, capsules and teas — and gained as rapidly as I lost.' *Plus ca change* is really all I can say to that!

The discovery of a chemical, DNTP, which raised the body's metabolism — and temperature — led to a rash of diet products and drugs containing it, despite the fact that it was literally deadly, causing many deaths as well as blindness and deafness. The American Medical Association announced in 1929 that every single item on the market was found to be dangerous or worthless. 'The desire to be slender,' it said, '— and slender to a degree often far beyond that compatible with good health — caused thousands of women to throw away money on so-called reduction treatments . . . '. Sound familiar? There were a number of deaths among prominent celebrities, which together with the A.M.A.'s warning brought a demand for a safe diet, giving rise to the first of the famous 'fad' diets, the Mayo diet, consisting of tomato juice and hard-boiled eggs. The A.M.A. retaliated by bringing out the first official diet. This was very unsound nutritionally, consisting of six bananas and four glasses of skimmed milk a day, with vegetable roughage to prevent constipation. The British, who were as weight-conscious by this time (the mid-thirties) as the Americans, eagerly followed similar regimes for losing weight. Periods of rationing during and after the war saw a relaxation in obsessive body-watching. Then one day I opened a newspaper and saw what was to be the start of the most diet-crazed period in history with its concomitant increase in fat prejudice. [1]

I am the same age as Twiggy, and it was at my most vulnerable time that the sixteen-year-old model burst upon the scene, sweeping away the lingering curves of the 1950s and exciting a whole New Look. The current obsession with size has mushroomed from that point in the 1960s, bringing with it a whole new armoury of diets, fitness plans and obsessions, not now with 'slimness', but with 'thinness'. I am a child of the 1960s — of the revolution against the Establishment, the quest for peace and not war, love and not hate. I marched with CND to Aldermaston and I sat in Trafalgar Square singing 'We Shall Overcome'. Along with so many others of my generation, the Beatles and Joan Baez were my idols, and Vietnam was my grief. I was a hippy, a Flower Child, a seeker of idealism in California. 'Make love, not war', ran the slogan so frowned upon by the generation above mine. It was called the Permissive Society and not without reason. The war and post-war taboos on sex and drugs were disappearing like snow in sunshine. It really did seem, in the 1960s, that the freedom of the individual was paramount. I can hear Neil Diamond, in the beautiful soundtrack from the film 'Jonathan Livingstone Seagull' singing, so poignantly, a song simply entitled 'Be'.

It seemed that the pervading exhortation to 'Be' which was truly the stamp of the golden decade did not include being fat. Every era has its heroines and heros and cult figures, and unlike previous decades where young people looked up to stars and singers who tended to be older, the Beautiful People of the 1960s were young teenagers and early twenties, and we wanted to be able to identify with them. As well as Twiggy, we had Cathy McGowan, who presented a hugely popular television pop music programme called *Ready Steady Go!* We had barefoot Sandie Shaw, the singer, and Jane Asher and Marianne Faithfull. They attracted a tremendous following of teenage girls who emulated them with their mini skirts, long straight hair and fringes. They were all thin with long legs. And for us in the 1960s they were the essence of womanhood.

Dieting became an obsession for many women. It became a virtually compulsory discipline, a commitment. It may have been a coincidence that the second Vatican Council of the Catholic Church — which had convened in the early sixties — had relaxed the rules about fasting and other disciplines loosely grouped under the heading of 'mortification of the flesh', and that fasting became part of a new spiritual discipline adopted by many people who had no relationship with the Catholic Church. While there is only a minority of Catholics in Britain, and a strong current of feeling against its doctrines, it does elicit a response from many, albeit a negative one. But the response tends to be strong, not indifferent. At the same time as our Western Church was moving away from fasting, so the same emphasis on purification by denial was being brought to us from the East by the Beatles and others who had heard teachings of an altogether new spiritual ideology. It may be that there is inbuilt into us a need for this kind of purging, and at a time of the loosening of sexual controls, some people unconsciously felt a need to tame the flesh in another direction. It was around this time that the 'slimmers' disease', anorexia nervosa, was fully identified; another means of fasting.

Minimum consumption of food during this time took on a sort of idealism. It was commonplace to miss breakfast and fashionable to eat grapefruit and drink black coffee. Artificial sweeteners became part of the contents of women's handbags, and it is rare today to find a woman under fifty who takes sugar in coffee or tea.

Hard as it is to imagine now, many newspapers and magazines during the 1950s and early 60s carried an advertisement for a product called 'Wate On', which had a line drawing of a curvaceous woman and an assurance that you, too, could look like that if you were too thin. I remember it clearly because I so envied those women who presumably thought they needed to buy the stuff. But the advertisement disappeared and was replaced by a fast blossoming array of private doctors and clinics who offered 'painless' aids to weight loss — a combination, in fact, of amphetamines (speed) and diuretics, together with a diet sheet. Jackie, a large Jewish woman, now sixty-five had battled all her life with a body naturally inclined to plumpness and a mother who insisted that she lose weight. For Jackie, the Harley Street diet doctors seemed the answer:

> You were given a diet sheet — I remember that you had to eat grapefruit before and after every meal and lots of meat. Then the pills to help you lose weight, though of course you weren't told what they were. You went back every week to be weighed and if you hadn't lost enough you were given a higher dose of amphetamines. When I reached my target weight I rang the clinic and was told to discontinue the pills but stick to the diet. The first evening I was tense and irritable and craved the pills. The next day I had gained several pounds — as a result of stopping the diuretics. I discovered that some women could not give up the amphetamines, they were really addicted. The whole process ruined my metabolism for life — the amphetamines speed up your whole body so much that when you stop them everything slows right down and you put on far more weight than you lost. I did, and have never been able to lose it.

With the increasing emphasis on weight loss came the beginnings of the health food movement, though in the 1960s and even early 70s it was still regarded as fairly cranky. Vegetarianism was bracketed with Eastern mysticism and regarded as an extension of spiritual discipline rather than a healthy way of eating. The first and best-known restaurant to open around that time was not called 'Cranks' for nothing. Just round the corner from

Carnaby Street it catered for the new wave of young people becoming conscious of the planet and its resources, of the cruelty to animals perpetrated so that we could eat meat and of the alternatives, in the form of a healthy vegetarian diet.

The majority view, though, was that vegetarianism was only for cranks and that fitness could not be achieved or maintained without plenty of meat, fish, cheese and eggs. After the leanness of the war years, it is perhaps understandable that high (animal) protein for health was preached as the food gospel. Those who wanted to lose weight were urged to eat as much as they liked in the meat, fish, cheese and eggs groups, together with vegetables and fresh fruit, but to give up those twin evils, bread and potatoes. And of course I did it myself. Being fat means having an ear unconsciously and automatically alert for every word pronounced about food, diet and weight loss. The poor potato has long since been accepted back into diet regimes, and since the high fibre recommendations, bread is seen to be essential. It is still possible to hear people say they are cutting out bread and potatoes to lose weight, so hard was that piece of wisdom drummed into us.

I started seriously dieting at thirteen. Looking back at those long, school photographs I see that it was not paranoid imagination that made me convinced I was the only fat girl in the school. I really was, though there were others *inclined* to be large. There was just one other girl, and she was in my year but she wasn't as fat as me, and though I willed her to put on weight so that I might have a companion in my isolation she lost it. Compulsory school medicals, which included weighing of course, brought the matron's wrath down upon my head. She demanded that I diet and completely refused ever to give me anything like sympathy on the rare occasions I was ill or had an accident at school. It was all my fault for being overweight, wasn't it? She herself had one of those withy-like bodies that bend in the middle — which was encircled by her hand-span nurse's belt. She had a lean face, a hooked nose and a high whining voice. I didn't think I had any right to hate her for her cruelty, though secretly I did, because, after all, I was the one in the wrong for being fat. So I was led to believe.

So surrounded by her threats, the jeers of my peer-group and the anxious encouragement of my friends I learnt about dieting, calorie counting, self-denial and the miseries of low blood sugar. I craved sugar so much that I could not bring myself to give it up in my tea which looking back is not really surprising. So deducting that from my daily calorie allowance (I drank a lot of tea) meant that I had to go without lunch and eat a diet supper. For some reason I insisted on white fish, green beans and steamed tomatoes and would eat no variation on that, for fear I might be beguiled into something 'forbidden'. This was the start of a lifetime of dieting — the cause of my weight now.

My mother was a doubtful collaborator. She could not ignore my misery at being outcast, so she prepared my fish and beans while at the same time urging me to have something else. Then every so often the sight of me coming home from school, weak and disorientated with low blood sugar, would rouse in her the fierce maternal urge to feed me. She knew one sure-fire way of getting me to break my diet and it always seemed to coincide with times when I myself felt I could go on no longer. So at those times I would come home to a bag of doughnuts, the only food I really could not resist — not one or two, but four or five, from the village bakery; soft and gooey, jammy and sugary. Then she would make me eat a proper supper — usually a pie of some sort, or stew and dumplings. The inexpressible comfort of being allowed to eat those things my body so craved after the bleak periods of starvation has left me with a permanent inability to resist a doughnut or anything with pastry round it, so bound up are those foods with memories of feeling satisfied and somehow returned to the world. But it was a yo-yo process because after the first joyful free days of having given up dieting I was back with the internal misery of not conforming and my fierce resolve to lose weight *once and for all* would begin all over again. I had started the diet-binge cycle.

The new massive slimming food industry had arrived. I used to buy a box of Limmits — delicious biscuits, two of which were 'a complete slimmers' meal'. They were supposed to contain all the essential nutrients but nothing could alter the fact that after eating them you felt as full as if you had eaten any two biscuits. Even then, I queried the advantage of eating my calories in this totally unsatisfying form, when I could have put together a reasonably filling meal for the same number of calories, or even — whisper who dares — have eaten a Mars Bar. But no, for the dedicated dieter, the purchase of a 'slimming' food showed a commitment to serious intentions about dieting. The fact was that I would eat my two Limmits — my complete meal — then feel so hungry, tastebuds awoken by their sweet, satisfying flavour, that I would proceed to eat the other four in the box, supposed to be a whole day's meals. But I was not able to exist on six biscuits a day.

Meanwhile specialist diets were appearing on the scene, each claiming to have the answer. There was the Scarsdale Diet, the Stillman Diet, the Mayo Clinic Diet, the Beverley Hills Diet. They were all high protein or high fat diets which counted calories. The dieting experts still agreed on one thing — carbohydrates were out. There was even a revolutionary very high fat diet, published in a book called *Eat Fat and Grow Slim*. Women's magazines and the Sunday papers published new, eccentric diets each week. People cut out the page and religiously followed instructions. The thing about these diets was that they used exactly the same basis as all the others, from the exotic film stars' Beverley

Hills diet to the unpalatable Mayo Clinic Diet which involved eating large numbers of boiled eggs. They all relied on cutting calories, and if you cut calories you lose weight, no matter what diet you follow. You can do it with any type of food — for example why not try the Delicious Doughnut Diet and lose weight fast!

Breakfast — cup of black coffee or tea, half a grapefruit with sugar substitute, thin piece of wholemeal bread or toast smeared with low-fat spread and Marmite, if liked.

Elevenses — cup of black coffee or tea and a sticky, sugary, jammy, FATTENING doughnut!

Lunch — poached egg on spinach, small slice of melon. No-cal drink (Cola, etc.) or black coffee or tea.

Tea — another doughnut!

Supper — two ounces white fish, large salad with lettuce, chopped raw cabbage, celery, tomato, chives, mint and parsley. Dress with tarragon vinegar.

Later in the evening — hunger pangs? Finish off the day with a cup of black coffee and comfort any first day dieting blues with YET ANOTHER doughnut! And you can eat three more tomorrow.

I've just made that up but the purpose of it is just to show that we can easily be seduced by diets, especially if they contain something nice to eat. An added enticement is seeing it all written down for you, so that if you just follow the diet sheet not only will you lose weight but you will be freed from the twin headaches of watching what you eat, calorie counting in other words, and constantly trying to work out menus for yourself. The Doughnut Diet will work because it contains approx 1100 calories. It also answers the question that used to puzzle me such a great deal, so conditioned are we to the idea of 'forbidden' foods. I could never work out why some people ate all sorts of fattening foods and did not put on weight. The answer is manifold of course, and consists of factors like individual metabolism and glandular activity. But it is also a fact that some people just do not want to eat very much and their daily calorie intake is often that of a dieter's even though they may be eating doughnuts!

More important is the fact that numerous studies have shown that some people do eat a great number of high-calorie foods, such as doughnuts and chocolate, and their weight remains constant. I am a good hearty eater but when I spent a recent week with a slim friend, I was amazed at the amount she could eat. A New Zealander, she was having none of this nonsense about cutting out butter or animal fats and I had glorious meals. (It is very satisfying to eat food with a high fat content when you have spent years on a low-fat, high-fibre regime as I have!) My grown-up daughters also eat a great deal and both love chocolate. There is a kind of perversity about the way they are complimented when anyone else sees them eating; people say things with great admiration like: 'Aren't you marvellous being able to eat all that and still stay slim!' as though my daughters could take the credit for their metabolisms and genetic predispositions not to gain weight. But as Llewellyn Louderback says in *Fat Power:* 'It's one of those psychological, fool-the-eye things. A fat person munching on a single stalk of celery looks gluttonous, while a skinny person wolfing down a twelve-course meal simply looks hungry.'[2]

And so diets and diet books have flourished. As far as the women's magazines approach to diet is concerned I have always been intensely irritated by those 'before and after' pictures — even more so when they have been used to advertise a particular diet product. The before pictures always show a woman slouching, badly dressed, with unkempt hair and suicidal expression on her face. It is impossible to see how much weight, if any, has been lost, when she is depicted standing straight and tall (presumably heavily corseted for maximum impact!) with a glad smile and a new hair-do. Even so, there are plenty of cases where women have lost five or six stones, or even more, and really do become almost unrecognizable. And of course there are the Slimmers of the Year — always someone who has lost a gargantuan amount, very quickly.

I have always been told when embarking on a diet that this must be a new way of eating, not just to lose the weight I needed to, but FOR LIFE. I agreed to that. It was worth it — to be freed of the stigma of being fat, to be fitter and to be able to move faster, not to have the nagging worry underlying my whole life that I was laying up trouble for myself in the form of all the life-threatening diseases which were the punishment for being fat — heart disease, high blood pressure, fatty arteries, diabetes. To remain on a diet seemed a small price to pay for all those benefits.

And yet I never could keep it up; and as 50 per cent of British women are a dress size 16 and over,[3] it seemed that I was not the only one. What made everything worse, as every dieter knows, is that when I broke my diets — even though I tried to 'watch what I ate' — then not only did I put the weight back on but more besides. So that in effect, I became heavier with each diet and yet was driven by social and medical pressure to keep trying again and again. It reminds me of the treadmill hospitals use to test your fitness, not only because of the analogy that you are working hard and yet getting nowhere but because of the effects of staying on that treadmill; the longer you stay on it, the less efficiently you perform, getting slower and disheartened until you collapse with exhaustion. The difference with the dieting treadmill though, is a fear many women have that if they *do* get off it their weight will shoot up. They find themselves with visions of weighing thirty stones (450lb) — or more — if they don't keep trying to diet, because once they are aware of their own capacity for gaining weight, it is logical to suppose there is no upper limit. The nightmare fantasy that creates sends them back to the diet books, even though they may ask the question that if they haven't been able to lose weight and keep it off in ten, twenty or thirty years, why should it be any different now?

1983 saw the publication of two new theories about diet and dieting. The Royal College of Physicians published its report on obesity which stated clearly that all the old dieting ideas about cutting out carbohydrates were wrong.[4] It recommended a high intake of unrefined carbohydrates and advocated wholemeal bread and pasta, cereals and potatoes in the diets of those trying to lose weight as well as those who were not. The old bread and potato taboo was finally lifted — officially. The word 'fibre' was suddenly high profile, and anyone interested in healthy eating knew that refined sugars/starches were bad news.

DIET BOOKS

Perhaps because of its official medical backing this wholefood way of eating was not regarded as cranky, as it had been twenty years before. It became fashionable to cook with brown rice, to eat brown bread, and to bake it too, and proprietary brands of breakfast cereal were heralded by a spate of wholesome, country-style television commercials. Meat-eating declined dramatically, especially red meat-eating, and pulses and beans appeared not only in wholefood stores but in village shops, a reliable indicator of any change in a nation's eating habits. Men were slower to take to this change, perhaps feeling that red meat fuelled red-blooded virility, and vegetarian cook books like *Not Just a Load of Old Lentils* were answered by cult-type titles such as *Real Men Don't Eat Quiche*, a statement fully endorsed by many men I have talked to who don't feel they have eaten a 'proper' meal unless they have a substantial portion of meat. In spite of their protests, the high fibre/wholefood diet appealed to women and it was not long before a new-wave slimming diet based on this kind of food appeared: Audrey Eyton's *F-Plan Diet* which claimed to be 'Quite simply, a phenomenon . . . more effective than any other slimming diet to date'.

It was a tempting diet, revolutionary in its use of bread, pasta, rice and cereal, with lovely filling-sounding recipes. It worked temporarily for thousands of people. The book of the F-Plan diet has been into countless reprints and Audrey Eyton has become a wealthy woman. I tried the F-Plan. It worked for me, too. Yet here I am today, heavier than ever. The Royal College of Physicians' Obesity Report stated that recidivism — gaining back weight lost — was something that happened to 95 per cent of dieters.[5] Some nutritionists put the figure as high as 98 per cent. No-one was saying dieting did not work — but something seemed to be happening that made it work only in the short term.

The second of the revolutionary new theories that exploded onto the diet scene in 1983 was formulated by nutritionist Geoffrey Cannon in a book with a title guaranteed to make weary dieters stop in their tracks and take notice. It was called *Dieting Makes You Fat*.[6] Geoffrey Cannon had developed from 'a plump little chap' into an overweight adult, who like so many of us had tried all the diets going and always regained weight. In the late 1970s he realized that his weight was staying constant, though he was eating and drinking whatever he wanted. The difference in his life-style was that he had taken up running. On a visit to Stanford University, California he learnt of a new medical discovery made by the Heart Disease Prevention Programme Unit there. The team had found the value of aerobic exercise — the kind where the heart and lungs are working strenuously for regular periods of twenty minutes or so at a time. Not only was this kind of exercise beneficial to the heart, but it actually increased the metabolic rate not just during the period of exercise but for about twenty-four hours afterwards.

Cannon went on to do his own research and discovered studies on metabolism that showed that dieting slows the basal metabolic rate by putting the body in a state of emergency, preparing it to store its reserves for famine. After a while, the system rebels at having to exist on fewer calories than is natural and the dieter feels longings for food which cause the return to normal eating, or bingeing — the body's protest at a long period of denial. As the basal metabolic rate has been lowered to prepare for famine, it will now require only (say) 2800 calories on which to function, instead of, for instance the 3000 it was accustomed to. If dieting is repeated, as it nearly always is, the metabolic rate gets slower each time, the reason for the weight loss-weight gain. Strenuous aerobic exercise is the answer to this, says Cannon; fast walking, swimming, running and a general move away from the lazy, sedentary twentieth-century life-style.

Cannon's book, *Fat to Fit*[7] is one of the few reasonable slimming books I have seen. He goes into detail about the quality of food required to be healthy and lose weight, he urges the use of homemade food full of nutrients, and with the use of ingenious wheel shaped diagrams shows how a balanced wholefood diet will provide all the ingredients we need. His eating plan is challenging and delicious and he begs the reader to dispense with calorie-counting, although he does give the calorie value of his meals, many of them coming out at around 700 calories each, over 2000 a day which is a mind-blowing thought for any dieter, conditioned to eat 700-1000 calories in order to lose weight.

I do think he is right. So why am I not doing it? Why aren't we all doing it? In my case the idea of that commitment to exercise terrifies me. I've done the twenty minute fast walk every day with evangelistic zeal, going out at midnight of course, so that no one could see me. And it didn't work. Years of being overweight have eaten away at my lower vertebral discs and I can't walk very far. A week of twenty minute brisk walks and my back seizes up and I can't move. So there's swimming. Not so easy with a full-time job and a pool twelve miles away, and the knowledge that this exercise, once started, is a lifetime commitment. I do agree with Geoffrey Cannon about the results of poor nutrition and the toll that calorie cutting takes on the body. But like stopping a diet, stopping the exercise will have the same effect — recidivism. I heard a radio discussion during which Cannon's 'dieting makes you fat' thesis was discussed. One doctor said he was threatening to write a book called 'Exercise Makes You Fat'. I knew what he meant. You cannot afford to stop it once started. At least taking exercise is an active way to lose weight and therefore psychologically more positive than the negative acts of denial that go with dieting. I may not have the willpower or stamina to attempt Cannon's vigorous exercise regime, but having dieted for thirty years I've learnt that the increasingly slowed metabolism theory is right. Calories may count, but I am not prepared to embark on a programme that will only allow me about 700 (which would make me lose weight) only to find that next time, after I have slipped off course, I can only lose weight on 650 — and so on.

And yet the diet books still try to hook us. I was surprised to find the *Independent* newspaper so taken in by *The Rotation Diet* by Martin Katahn[8] — that it pronounced it the Independent Diet of the Decade. It sounds a good idea when you first read it, if you *can* read it without hurling it across the room, so smug and patronising is Katahn's style. Basically you diet for three weeks on a very low calorie intake — 600-900 for two of the weeks with one week on 1200. The week on 1200 calories is very important, stresses Katahn, or you will reduce your metabolic rate — he acknowledges the starvation response without acknowledging that a long-dieted body is likely to reduce its metabolic rate on his plan, too.

With the fervour of a Southern Baptist, Katahn tells us that the average weight loss in twenty-one days was twelve and a half pounds. This is not particularly outstanding when you consider that for two thirds of that time you have only been allowed to eat 600-900 calories. But here comes the treat, the thing that makes *this* diet different (I feel weary at this point; haven't we heard it all before?). After three weeks, you *stop dieting*. Katahn assumes that it will be very hard to do so and in many cases he may be right. Low calorie rapid weight loss can make some people feel 'high' with success, but the break is necessary for several reasons: to increase motivation, to ensure there is no reduction in metabolic rate, to learn the practice of maintenance. I had finished reading the section on the break from dieting without finding anything that suggested that dieting had stopped. That was because it had not. The 'break' after three weeks simply means that you can eat more calories — but they still have to be carefully counted. Women, while 'not dieting', can eat between 1200 and a dizzy 1800 calories a day, *as long as they are taking forty-five minutes brisk exercise every day.* Then after any time between a week or a month, you go back on the old 600-900 regime.

Nowhere in this book can I find Katahn's carrot — a break from dieting — put into practice. His nutritional knowledge is sound and he has climbed onto the bandwagon of essential daily exercise but after all that, he is just another calorie counter. I am not sure how many women could stomach his use of language which suggests that he and the reader know what a wicked, bad thing food is 'but together we can beat it'. His book is full of words and phrases that sound to me as though he regards food as having the same destructive potential as an unexploded bomb. On his diet we may have unlimited 'free vegetables', and for those times when temptation threatens, then we can fall back on the 'safe fruit' of our choice, but only *one* kind of fruit, mind. This safe fruit is the answer to all dieting difficulties, and Katahn imparts this secret in type heavy with italics, and capital italics, giving the whole thing a conspiratorial feel. So if you choose grapefruit, as he himself has, make sure it is always in the house, or with you at work. Because:

Every time you get the urge to deviate from the Rotation Diet you reach for your safe fruit. Believe me, it's a charm! It's your absolute guarantee of success. It beats the complete failure that occurs when you allow yourself to dip into the sweet jar or biscuit tin, begin to feel disgusted with yourself for having blown your diet and then let all hell break loose . . . Use it . . . as an insurance or 'fallback' food to be used whenever it is needed to prevent *dangerous deviations* (my italics) from the Rotation Diet.

Hallelujah! With this diet surely we shall all be saved. Praise the Lord! But the road to salvation is the straight and narrow one, isn't it? No room on it for fatties. So what must I do to be saved, Mr Katahn?

> You must make a decision to be absolutely perfect in following the Rotation Diet. PERFECT? That word frightens you, doesn't it? . . . I suspect that you may have had too many failures in the past to trust yourself on any plan that calls, from the start, for perfection . . . After you see what the diet requires, as well as the exercise programme, *you must take about half an hour to sit down and plan how to be perfect.*

The book continues in that vein, reinforcing the idea that fat is bad by the repeated use of such words as success, failure, deviation, temptation, danger, permissible, allowable, forbidden.

Those of us who are overweight have choices to make and decisions to face about whether or not to attempt to lose weight in a way that will be permanent. The years of failed dieting and regained weight hardly serve as encouragement and the question we have to ask ourselves is: 'If I have failed to lose weight permanently up till now, what magic factor is going to make it work next time?' It becomes a depressing vicious circle, where feelings spiral round: I want to lose weight once and for all; this time it will be different with X new diet and an exercise plan; but it has never worked before; do I really want to lose weight? why can't I accept myself as a fat woman? why can't other people accept my fat? But even if I make the choice to stay fat and learn to love my fat self, I am at risk medically, so they tell me, from all those things like high blood pressure and heart disease. I don't want to risk my health so I will have to lose weight effectively, once and for all; but how?

One thing is certain; the answer does not lie in diet books, however convincing they sound, or however novel their approach. They are all flawed. Rosemary Conley is the woman whose name is almost synonymous with dieting in the 1990s. Among the hundreds of diet books published every year in Britain, her first book stood out and hooked women in the area they are often most vulnerable. It was called *The Hip and Thigh Diet* and it sold a million copies. Women — British women in particular — have a terror of being 'pear-shaped', of being the shape, in fact, that makes us differ from men who tend to be rounded all over — 'apple-shaped'. The extra fat on women's hips and thighs is biological, but most women hate it. And although anyone who stops to think knows that spot-reducing — targeting a specific part of your body for weight loss — is one of dieting's long disproven myths, women turn a blind eye. It seems to be symbolic of their desperation to achieve the androgynous model's body, to do away with the visible signs of fertility that are signified by wideness of hips and thighs.

Rosemary Conley capitalised on her success by following her first book with *The Complete Hip and Thigh Diet*, then the *Inch Loss Plan*, the *Metabolism Booster Diet* and *The Whole Body Programme*. I do wonder why people don't ask the obvious question — if one diet *really* works, the author does not need to write books on others! And what has *The Complete Hip and Thigh Diet* got that the plain old *Hip and Thigh Diet* has not?! Conley now has eight books and videos on sale and all are bestsellers. Her knowledge of eating and weight is in my opinion unsound and she makes the common mistake of associating fat with overeating despite at least 20 studies that indicate that this is not so. 'Bingeing, is I believe, the greatest cause of overweight', she writes, and that overweight must be the result of 'too many fatty and sugary foods which are positively loaded with calories — bread spread with lashings of butter, an abundance of fried foods, cream cakes, biscuits, chocolates, crisps and so on. The types of food overweight people love.' The types of food *many* people love and many do not, whether they are fat or thin, but Rosemary Conley buys into the stereotype of the fat person gorging herself. You can always identify believers in this stereotype and the implicit disparagement that goes with it, by their reference to 'cream cakes'. Not fruit cakes or sponge cakes, but the type that are linked in the public consciousness with fat people's eating habits.

Challenged on Britain's hard-hitting *Dispatches* programme on Channel 4,[9] Rosemary Conley's wide smile did not leave her face. 'I'm actually making people healthier and they look better,' was her opinion.

The experts gave their views. Professor Kelly Brownell of Yale said: 'Preposterous! . . . This is again an example of "What do people want, what will they buy, what they want is . . . so let's write *The Hip and Thigh* book". A spokesman from the British Heart Foundation was concerned about the excessive claims being made for diets. The Foundation has produced a 'Factfile' for GPs warning them of the dangers. *The Hip and Thigh Diet* is not recommended. There is also no such thing as 'metabolism boosting'. Rosemary Conley's reply to the experts was: 'What I'm saying is that if you have got excess fat in that area (hips and thighs) you will lose it from there first; if you've got excess weight around your tummy or bust you'll also lose it from there first. So I think they basically haven't understood what I'm trying to say.'

Nor did I after that complicated statement. Rosemary Conley's nutrition is reasonably sound — her diet is low fat, though she 'forbade' oily fish, which has long since been known to have a beneficial effect on the heart. However, this has apparently been pointed out to her, and she will include it in her updated books. But you didn't need a diet book to tell you that in the first place.

As a book reviewer for a woman's magazine I get diet books by the score. I can see my bookshelf from here with its gimmicky contents — the *Two Day Diet, The 35 Plus Diet, The Only Diet There Is, Eat Yourself Thin*. Almost anyone could write a successful diet book (successful in terms of sales, I mean!). You just need to bone up on nutrition (minimally), calories, the 'dangers' of being fat, the joys of being slim, think of a different formula and away you go. How about the *Fat Woman's Diet Book*? The fact is that diet books are just another branch of the vast, profit-grabbing, exploitative slimming industry, as are slimming magazines. Perhaps surprisingly, there are more slimming magazines in Britain than America, and there are none in Germany, for instance.

WHAT DIETING HAS DONE TO EATING

When we diet we seem to enter a tunnel of existence in which the only real focus of concentration is what we have eaten, should eat, should not have eaten and how many calories we have consumed, pounds lost, inches disappeared in the mist. Our lives are bounded with tape measures and scales and diet books. In short, we start dieting and stop living.

The Minnesota study, conducted by nutritionist and physiologist Professor Ancel Keys is a startling example of this. Young, healthy conscientious objectors volunteered to live in the University of Minnesota for six months towards the end of World War II. The aim was to monitor the effects of deprivation, with war-torn Europe in mind, and the participants were given a diet similar to that of the victims of war.[10] For the first three months the group of thirty-six men ate normally while their behaviour, eating patterns and personality were studied. Then for three months they were put on strict diets with their normal intake cut by half, followed by a further three month period where they began to eat normal amounts of food again. They had never had any previous interest in either food or diets.

The effects were significant. Food became the main topic of conversation, reading and daydreams for almost all the men. About two-thirds of them who had had no previous interest in cookery became fascinated by it and began to read cookery books and to collect recipes. About half way through the period of semi-starvation thirteen of the men expressed an interest in taking up cooking when the experiment was over. A few even planned to become chefs. Many of the men found it impossible to keep to the diet, eating secretly and then feeling guilty. They worried more and became more prone to depression, they found difficulty in concentrating and began to withdraw from others. Their personalities returned to normal after the semi-starvation period, but a good many of them had eating problems, wanting more food than they were given and being preoccupied with the food and how they would eat it. They lost their sense of appetite and satiety, some developed cravings for certain foods, and some developed an over-awareness of their weight and went on another reducing diet. The physical and psychological effects of the experiment lasted for up to eight months after it was over.

Historical and cultural studies of dearth and famine have consistently shown that deprivation *changes* the psychology and personality of human beings. Even if the essential nutrients are present, calorie restriction produces dramatic results. Dieters — voluntary or otherwise — experience fatigue, depression and irritability. The ability to concentrate declines, all creative power and achievement is affected. The obsession with food is ever-present and some people even veer towards psychosis.

When I was a fat, unhappy teenager, permanently on and off diets and trying to work for exams, I remember periods of complete inability to study or concentrate, when I would read the same passage over and over without it making sense, when I would stare at a blank sheet of paper, pen in hand. It was not a case of not understanding the subject, it was more like pathways in my brain not linking together

— I knew what to do but I couldn't make my brain do it. My mother, noticing these periods, would intervene. 'What you need is a square meal inside you, my girl' she would say, and despite my protests she would cook me one of her meat and vegetable pies with all the trimmings. 'No more of that white fish and green beans nonsense' she'd announce firmly, and of course there was no way my starving self could resist the aroma of real food which was put before me while she stood to make sure I ate it. She knew nothing of the research, had no academic knowledge of the effects of dieting, but she was right. Eating a good meal with enough calories enabled me to study, to write essays and to wonder why I had not been able to do it in the first place. Chilling, therefore, to read that at the time of the *Pueblo* crisis, President Johnson was reported to be on a rigid 350 calories per day diet:[11] And to wonder about others, men and women, upon whose authority and judgement the entire world depends.

Dieting takes away the social meanings of eating, and prevents the unifying and bonding effects of sharing food with others. Anna Knowles[12] tells a moving story of a journey she took in Greece, in a rickety old bus 'full of peasants with bundles and parcels. Our fellow passengers were shy, but intrigued by two foreigners with back-packs and maps. Hesitantly they unwrapped their bundles.' Anna Knowles says she is still moved to tears at this bridge between strangers and cultures, created by the simple act of the Greeks unwrapping their bundles and inviting them to share their parcels of rough bread, cheese and olives. Her first instinct was to refuse, knowing how poor they were, but then she saw the significance of the gesture. The scraps of food were

powerful emblems of hospitality and generosity made all the more precious by the poverty of our benefactors.

So we broke bread with strangers and in doing so we crossed barriers of language, of culture and nationality and became their friends.

Anna Knowles also says that if you are watching every mouthful you eat you will be presented with a dilemma if you want to participate in the spontaneous sharing of food: you can be hemmed in and restricted, preoccupied with every mouthful and with the satisfaction of a trim figure; or you can accept that the pleasure of friendship and a sociable life-style will make you gain weight.

When I had lunch with Ken Hom, the Chinese-American cook, I commented that he was missing out on the chatter going on amongst the guests (he was cooking the meal at somebody's house). His reply assured me that he was not missing out at all; on the contrary he felt privileged to be the one doing the cooking. 'Cooking a meal for someone is one of the most intimate, physical things you can do for them,' he told me. 'Food is like sex. You reach out and touch people with food.' He went on to describe various 'eating tours' he had been on all over China, where the preparation and sharing of food was of paramount importance in forming social bonds between people. In one poor region of south-west China he had attended a goat banquet. Fifty-five courses had been served, all prepared from goat, so that every part of the animal was eaten. The emphasis was on using and not wasting food. Dieting was unheard of.

Anthropologist Margaret Mackenzie says that 'In all societies, eating is absolutely a central focus of meanings. Whether those meanings be restraint or pleasure or joy or familial connection or relation to the sacred or relation to other people, eating will always embody those meanings. A mistake weight reduction programs make is that you can't leach all meanings out, no matter how much you try.'[13]

Food is highly symbolic, from the obligatory consumption of sheep's eyes in some Eastern countries, so as
not to offend the host, to the food that accompanies rites
of passage, some of which we still observe in the West, like
Christening feasts, weddings and to a certain extent
funerals, though the old idea of a wake where people ate
and remembered the deceased with thanksgiving for her or
his life is largely obsolete in England. We still eat at
celebrations like Christmas or Thanksgiving in America,
but the pleasure is marred by constant exhortations to diet
before or after the event to lose the pounds that we are sure
to gain during it. In her book *The Hungry Self* Kim Chernin
talks of a new rite of passage for young women — the
initiation at college into a collective ceremonial of bingeing
and vomiting.[14]

I have a close friend, Jewish, who embodies the essence
of Jewish womanhood — she has a compulsion to feed
people. It is wonderful going to her house because there is
always so much food and it is so *good*. I associate her with
feelings of well-being and comfort and a great sense of
being welcome. You cannot help feeling that when someone
presses something delicious onto you, bought or prepared
with generosity and love. She even has several stray cats
who moved in when they realized that to be seen around
her back door was to be fed. This friend tells me that the
British Telecom commercial where Maureen Lipman
opened a full-to-bursting fridge and bemoaned that she had
got no food in the house is typically Jewish and sums up
in a nutshell their feelings about food. I have been regaled
with stories of the foods prepared for Jewish celebrations
— food for the gods, says my friend. She glows with warmth
and open-heartedness. To turn from that to the coldness of
diets and diet books is to step from a warm house into the
chill night air.

The act of dieting takes the place of real living, placing

restraints not only on the dieter, but on friends and family. Actress Lynn Redgrave's autobiography makes this so clear. She describes a visit home to England from California where she now lives. Four weeks previously, she and her 12-year-old daughter had joined Weight Watchers (this comes in a chapter entitled 'Salvation' — the religious connection yet again). This was an important and moving visit to her family. Her father, actor Michael Redgrave, was frail and ill. Her parents had never seen Lynn's two-year-old daughter, Annabel. It was a meeting 'awash with love and family sentiment'. Her mother, actress Rachel Kempson, prepared an English tea with shortbread and treacle tart. Lynn and her daughter looked desperately in the larder for some carrots. Dinner divided the family; for her and her daughter there was: 'Steamed fish with lemon and a little ginger and a salad with local dressing on a night when Mum and Dad were tucking into beef bourguignon with potatoes mashed in almost a pound of Normandy butter'. The two-week stay was 'our toughest test yet'. How sad, it seems to me, to be in the grip of the tyranny of dieting during a rare and special visit home. After all, you do not gain weight from eating normal foods. She didn't have to have the pound of Normandy butter. And her steamed fish, carrots and salad regimen prevented her mother doing that age-old thing — cooking, with love, for her family to enjoy a meal together.

Lynn Redgrave says her eating was out of control before 'Salvation'. She was possessed, she says by something which she calls 'Fat Ogre' — a sort of demon. The following incident, which took place after she had joined Weight Watchers, sounds more hysterical than merely 'out of control'. Redgrave was on a plane, and although she was allowing herself three glasses of wine a week, 'I knew that a glass on board at this early stage of my eating retraining could be a disaster. The stewardess appeared. "Hi, Miss

Redgrave, my name is Kimberley. How are you today? . . . A little Chardonnay?" Her voice rapidly descended a couple of octaves, while her head seemed to spin madly round and round, *Exorcist* fashion. *"Fat Ogre" I scream silently, "I'd know you anywhere."* "Excuse me," I smiled tightly. "I have to go to the bathroom." How long had my Weight Watchers classmate said? Ten minutes? By the time I emerged fifteen minutes later, a line had formed outside the toilet but . . . at least for now, my Chardonnay crisis was over.'[15]

I think Lynn Redgrave is a tragic example of the life-diminishing, mind-narrowing effects of dieting. This book is her autobiography. She comes from one of the most famous and talented families of the century. She is a brilliant and successful actress and always has been — she was a founder member of the National Theatre Company in London. She has three children, and that rarity in show-business, a long and happy marriage. She has the gift of writing, not just well, but *beautifully*, though this is not apparent when she writes about weight and dieting. She has a fund of wonderful stories and anecdotes. Yet her book is called *Diet For Life: How I lost Weight and Learned to Stay Slim*. Half the book comprises Weight Watchers menus and recipes and the other half is more about Lynn Redgrave's weight than about the woman or the actress.

There is a pay-off of course. I have not forgotten that this chapter is about the diet industry. Celebrity spokespeople for the diet industry are *in*. The Celebrity Endorsements Network estimates earnings of $100,000 to $300,000 per year for the endorsements. Number one in the industry is Weight Watchers, with Lynn Redgrave promoting them since the early 1980s. Her appearances in their advertisements has boosted Weight Watchers food sales by 100 per cent.[16] The acknowledgements in her book begin with Foodways National, the Heinz Company and DDB Needham Worldwide Advertising Agency, and move on to various Weight Watchers personnel. And the jacket of the book is stamped with the Weight Watchers logo.

I was looking for an exam congratulations card when I found a card I had not seen before. It depicted a woman running, her face one broad grin, holding the waist of her trousers which ballooned out, about twenty sizes too big. Above the picture was the message: 'What a successful diet!' and inside the card: 'People will be seeing less of you now! Congratulations.'

This card conveyed a host of messages to me. It reinforced the achievement factor of losing weight, thus tacitly endorsing society's overview of the fat person as failure. And I found its message insidiously political, in the suggestion that people would be seeing less of the recipient. Fat people take up too much space. If we can't exterminate them, at least let's encourage them to destroy some of their body. Congratulations on disappearing! Exams and driving tests, giving birth, baptism, marriage and confirmation — there are congratulations cards for all of these and it is good that there are for they are rites of passage which deserve to be marked. The card that commemorates a milestone in your life resonates with memory and association when you take it out from an album or drawer and look at it years later.

Do you do that with a diet card? Especially when it is unlikely that the weight loss will be maintained? Why don't we have cards saying: 'Congratulations on having your hair cut. There will be a lot less of it to wash now'; or for the anorexic: 'Congratulations on your recovery. It's nice to see your curves again'.

The simple fact is that losing weight is big business and this crazy card just means that at least one card manufacturer has realized that there is money to be made out of a cultural obsession.

Pick up any women's magazine and the chances are that you will find somewhere in its pages an article which directly or in another context deals with weight loss. The reasons for this are two-fold and uncomplicated. First, most women want to lose weight, are fascinated by anything that promises them reduction, drawn to anything that will kill the hated flesh, dissolve it, chop it up and dispose of it. Every new diet and eating plan carries a message of hope because it is different: 'So you've never been able to lose weight before, but this is revolutionary' . . . and women are believers because they *want* to believe. It is the eternal Grail quest and magazines which are in touch with the latest medical and beauty developments may find the way for us. Underneath we all know the truth that diets do not work. But women's magazines are at the nerve-centre, will be the first to bring us the good news of our salvation. So articles about diet and weight loss by other means help sell women's magazines. I picked a handful at random and looked at the cover-lines, chosen as the features most likely to make women buy the magazine. My random sample proclaimed on their covers:

10 PAGE BODY SPECIAL — YOUR GUIDE TO A BETTER SHAPE

TOTAL FITNESS — THE EASY WAY

28 DAY DIET (THE ONE THAT KNOWS YOUR BODY)

FEELING FAT AND UNFIT? — HEALTH AND BEAUTY GUIDE THAT REALLY WORKS

SO YOU'RE PEAR SHAPED — FOUR WEEK ACTION PLAN THAT WORKS

WIN A WEEK AT A TOP HEALTH FARM

PAMPER YOURSELF AT A HEALTH HYDRO

DE-TOX DIET — A FAST FIX FOR FEELING FIT

FLATTEN YOUR STOMACH IN JUST FIVE
MINUTES A DAY

FAT SUCTION — HOW TO BUY YOURSELF THIN

DOES PLASTIC MAKE PERFECT — ONE WOMAN'S
COMPULSIVE QUEST FOR BEAUTY

WHAT WEIGHT WATCHERS TAUGHT ME — BY ITS
FOUNDER

WARNING — YOUR HUSBAND CAN MAKE YOU
FAT

And a rarity from the one magazine not afraid to speak out,
She magazine, the only one that accepted my feature which
eventually led to this book and which proclaimed on its
cover:

BEING FAT IS NOT A SIN — A PLEA FOR AN END
TO PREJUDICE[17]

So women buy magazines with a fascination for these
articles. But there is another reason why women's
magazines are so strong on fitness, shape and weight loss
and that is because of the advertisers. Many people think
that a magazine relies on obtaining its income from its cover
price. Not so, that is only a small proportion of the complex
financial structure and the mutually dependent relationship
between magazines and advertisers. If publications do not
get sufficient, main-line advertising they cannot afford to
produce themselves and they fold. The editorial policy of
a magazine is to a large extent answerable to its advertisers.
Women's magazines are big on the advertising of fashion,
beauty and food, but that generally means 'healthy' foods

and includes slimming foods or products that will appeal for their low calorie content. So magazines of this type literally cannot afford to promote in their features the sort of ideas that will antagonise their advertisers. Every magazine has its own 'image' and advertising is targeted towards that, because the type of woman who reads magazine A for its image and content is likely to buy the sort of goods advertised in its pages. If that magazine departs too far from its editorial policy then its readers will look for another that suits their lifestyle and aspirations and the advertisers will lose customers.

The trend in magazines now is towards more gloss, more style, better design, bright glowing covers. The message is be fit, but in the swim, don't hover on the edge of life, be up to the minute, fashionwise, beautywise, shapewise. Health is a big issue at the moment, not surprisingly in an age where killer diseases are rife and our wellbeing is under constant threat from the damage we do to the earth and ourselves by pollution of all kinds. And weight is part of the popular image of health.

Having worked on women's magazines I can vouch for the fact that they practise what they preach — editorial staff are invariably slim, well-groomed, fashion-conscious and ever watchful for the dreaded weight gain. It is a circular dance, involving the advertisers who dictate image, the magazines who promote it and the readers who respond to it taking their *modus vivendi* from the articles and buying the products which endorse what they have read about. This is the media pressure that fat people are up against, reproduced not only in newspapers and magazines but in television and film and especially television and film commercials which cost millions to make. These are often brilliant gems of theatre in miniature, so clever and sophisticated, not to mention subliminal, that it is difficult to ignore them and even more difficult to take a deliberate stance against what they so seductively sell.

Even though half of Britain's women are over size 16, the advertising and image-creating business is not responding except with tokenism. A friend who is a fashion editor on a well-known glossy told me that they were conceding to the now well-publicized statistic by extending their special offers to include a size 18, but she was reluctant about it. She felt that if women wanted fashionable clothes they should slim to fit them rather than designers and manufacturers having to create larger sizes and magazine offers to include them.

So magazines and advertisers are collaborators in the promotion of thinness and it suits both parties to do so. There is a massive industry making millions of pounds out of women's desire to be slim and that would go down the drain if magazines started to encourage women to relax about their weight. Specialist slimming magazines like *Slimmer* and *Weight Watchers* have no problems with advertising; they are a gold mine for the slimming industry. But the fact that there is no major magazine catering for the large numbers of women who want positive messages about being fat is significant. When Eleanor Graham started her privately owned *Extra Special* she had to work hard to find advertisers other than Evans and a few other large size clothes manufacturers. The magazine was a continuing financial headache for her and the fact that there is so little support from advertising revenue is the reason that there is no mainstream magazine for large women either here or in America. *Radiance*, the equivalent of *Extra Special* in the States runs on the same small budget for the same reasons, as does UK's *YES* and *Pretty Big*.

THE BRANDED PRODUCT MARKET

Where dieting is concerned there is often a feature or survey carried out in collaboration with a publication and manufacturer. For example, in 1988 *Cosmopolitan* ran a massive survey on health in conjunction with the makers of Outline, a low fat slimmers' margarine. In October 1988 the results were published and claimed to be 'one of the most comprehensive health surveys ever', taking up four pages of the magazine. The survey was concerned with all aspects of health, but of course it included weight and eating patterns. Results showed that on the whole readers' weight was on the low side, most weighing between 8½ and 9½ stones (120 and 133lb). Yet a staggering 78 per cent reported that they would like to lose weight; 66 per cent dieted spasmodically and 15 per cent were on permanent diets.

While not actively promoting the use of Outline spread, the survey reported that many readers had responded to the low, unsaturated fat publicity. Nearly two-thirds now used low fat spreads instead of butter. The message is subliminal: the endorsement of a survey on health by a product then leads to that product being associated in people's minds with good health.

This comforting association with health can be a trap for the diet-conscious unwary, a fact that was revealed in a survey of ready-prepared complete meals aimed at dieters and 'healthy eaters'. In May 1992, the British Food Commission's *Food Magazine* published a report in which the Coronary Prevention Group analysed 75 of these meals including Findus Lean Cuisine, Birds Eye Healthy Options and Heinz Weight Watchers. Sales of these reached £90 million in 1991.

With a healthy heart in mind, the Coronary Prevention Group looked at the content of fat, particularly saturated fat, fibre and salt. The Findus range passed the fat tests but nearly half the samples tested were low in fibre and carbohydrate and were too salty. Most of the Birds Eye meals were low in fibre, and some were high in saturates.

Five of the Heinz Weight Watchers meals tested had too much fat, three had too much *saturated* fat, all were salty and more than half had insufficient fibre. Boots Shapers ready meals came out badly too; half the sample had too much fat and only one had enough carbohydrate. One Heinz meal had a fat level of 44 per cent and one from Boots came out at 57 per cent. Of the 42 meals which claimed to be low in fat, only seven actually were. Also found guilty in the survey were own-brand meals from Tesco and Sainsburys. I noticed that very soon after this report came out there was a spate of new television commercials advertising these foods as new, improved, etcetera — some advertising agencies must have been burning the midnight oil!

In the July 1993 issue, the British consumer magazine *Which* reassessed branded diet products in an article whose title conveyed their findings: 'Diets that help you lose £££.' Meal replacements, they said, 'could prove to be a dieter's worst enemy as they don't tackle the eating habits that cause people to put on weight in the first place and, at worst, could lead to a physically and psychologically damaging cycle of weight loss and weight gain'. *Which* asked for evidence that these slimming plans work. Nestlé claimed to have evidence of long-term success but would not show this to the magazine.

The survey found that in spite of the 1992 Food Commission report, these meal replacements were still high in fat, sugar and calories and low in fibre. They were also extremely expensive. *Which* asked 25 people who had used meal replacement products to fill in a questionnaire. Most said they had tried them because they wanted to lose weight quickly and easily. But 15 of the 25 did not lose weight, and of the ten who did, five regained all the weight lost — and more — and two regained some of it.

A draft European Community (EC) directive has drawn up rules to control the claims and content of meal replacements. Products should not refer to the amount of weight that can be lost or to the speed of weight loss. All the plans examined by *Which* encouraged rapid weight loss. 'Slimfast', for example, (whose muesli bar, described as 'a healthy snack' contained 4g of fat, 12g of sugar and 110 calories in only 28g) claims to be 'the healthy way to lose weight fast' — a statement which, especially in the light of research documenting the dangers of fast weight-loss, is surely a contradiction in terms.

The EC draft says that an individual meal replacement should provide at least 200 calories — many have fewer and the Boots yogurt shake has only 99. The draft recommends the banning of claims that these replacements will make you feel less hungry or more satisfied. Only one plan tested did not make this claim. Under UK food labelling regulations, it must be made clear that these products should not replace all your meals and that your third meal should be highly nutritious.

An enormous variety of 'slimming' foods are available. These were useful for calorie-counters in the days before nutritional information, including calorie values, was stated on food packaging. Now there is no need to buy into the diet industry in this way. For one thing, it keeps the mind fixed in the narrow channel marked 'diet'. And if you really want to keep an eye on calories, buy ordinary, wholesome foods and check their nutritional content. Low-fat eating, whether dieting or not, is widely recommended and low-calorie preparations, such as for salad dressing can be useful. Try to avoid the ones sold as specific diet products.

Sue Dibb, co-director of the Food Commission, an independent body, said on *Dispatches*: 'The food industry is a powerful lobby and it is very intertwined with the slimming industry. Some scientists linked with the food industry are advising the government on health and nutrition.' The main watchdog body of experts which advises the Department of Health is the Committee on Medical Aspects of Food, or COMA. *Dispatches* found that as many as half of the 42 members of COMA panels have at some time undertaken paid work for companies involved in the food industry. Scientists depend largely on funding for their research so are reluctant to bite the hand that feeds them. And government policy is influenced by industry. A good example is the question of why cigarette advertising is not banned in Britain, since smoking is an acknowledged health hazard complete with Government health warnings.

The diet industry infiltrates even those places where you think you might get an independent opinion. A survey carried out for the National Dairy Council found that when asked for advice on diet, 71 per cent of nurses in doctors' surgeries gave out leaflets produced by the food industry.

REPLACEMENT MEALS

These have been around for a long time but women are still bewitched into parting with large sums of money to buy a calorie counted milk-shake, soup, biscuit or bar with which to replace one or two meals a day. These diet plans cleverly avoid coming under the maligned VLCD category (very low calorie diets) by suggesting you eat a 'normal' meal at least once a day. However, these replacement 'meals' only contain between 120-200 calories per serving, so two replacement meals would give you about 400 calories in total. If you then have the recommended 'normal' meal of 350-450 calories, you are still on considerably fewer than 1000 calories a day. And that is not enough.

I sent my 18-year-old daughter, Lindsay, (who has never dieted) to do some research for me on the latest calorie values and prices of these products. She went and stood at the appropriate counter in one of Boots the Chemist's large branches and was bewildered by the huge variety on offer.

As she stood with notebook and pen, she was even more puzzled, and at times highly amused, by the customers. She came back full of stories. First of all, she said, no-one who bought the products was fat, or could have been called overweight. What were they doing there? she wondered. She told me of one woman: 'She tottered over on stilettos, dragging her husband by the arm, saying "Come along, I've got to get a diet plan." She was really thin. Her husband was looking all puzzled and said to her "What are you talking about?" "A *diet* plan" said the woman. "Now which one shall I have?" "Who's it for?" said her husband, and she tapped his arm, as if to say, silly man! "For *me*, of course," she said. He just looked completely out of it and wandered off to look at the cameras!' Then there was the thin woman who stood for ages by Lindsay, looking at the range of products and sighing. In the end, she muttered 'It's got to be done' and resolutely picked up a drum of Slimfast.

My daughter found this all highly entertaining and amazing. But the power of the industry cannot be underestimated — it has most of the female population of Britain and the United States in its grip, under one guise or another. Television commercials are powerful motivators, showing the 'before' photographs, deliberately unflattering, with some bright, upbeat woman saying, in effect, can you really believe that awful disgusting creature was me? Then I discovered Waste Away (or whatever) and now look at me. There are the jingles and the clever graphics and women think — ah, there's the answer.

Moral of the story — don't do it. What is the point? You can eat a decent meal instead. You can eat a Mars Bar for 300 calories! The diet industry is *unethical* — don't buy into it. At a time of deepest recession, it is one of the few that seems completely immune. What an indictment of women's obsession.

After the low calorie meals and meal replacements, dieters

enter a minefield of pills, potions and VLCDs. In the pills and potions category come the tablets claiming to reduce your appetite and those which actually say they will reduce your weight. The appetite suppressants are based either on sugar or on a bulking agent which is designed to swell in the stomach, giving you a feeling of fullness. Before a meal, or indeed any time when you feel hungry, your blood sugar is low. The sugar based appetite suppressants give your blood sugar a short-term boost; a glucose sweet would do exactly the same thing. But the body produces insulin as a result of the sugar boost, and as a result blood sugar can drop as low as or lower than it was before you ate the product, making you hungrier than ever in a short time.

The bulking agents contain fibre, such as Branslim, or guar or locust bean gum, or other gums such as glucomannan, galactomannan and xanthan. They really do not have any effect on the appetite and the Ministry of Agriculture, Fisheries and Food is concerned that these gums may swell in the gullet, causing breathing problems. In the United States, one such product has been taken off the market after a five-year battle. The American Food and Drugs Administration reported 17 cases of obstruction in the oesophagus and one death as a result of surgery to remove the obstruction in the throat. The product, Cal–Ban 3000, had been dodging the authorities for years due to aggressive marketing techniques.

MAGIC PILLS AND POTIONS

Some of these make extraordinary claims, like the mail-order De-toxification diet plan. This declares that the body gets 'toxic build-up' and that the only way it can deal with it is to lock it away inside new fat cells. This is why, the blurb runs, some women say that dieting actually *makes* them fat!

There are a host of these 'magic' pills in Britain and even more in America, where the claims are often more outrageous: 'The Fat Blocker' can 'flush calories right out of the body'; 'Dream Away' advises 'Just take Dream Away before going to bed. You will wake up in the morning slimmer, trimmer'. Then there was the 'Fat Magnet' pill which was claimed to: 'break into thousands of particles, each acting like a tiny magnet, attracting and trapping many times its size in undigested fat particles ... then all the trapped fats and calories are naturally flushed out of the body.'[18] America's Federal Trade Commission took the manufacturers to court, asking for $5 million in refunds. Then there are the extraordinary teas, a real scam, promising weight losses of two and a half stones (35lb) in 29 days. As one consultant physician said — you could only lose that amount by amputating limbs!

There are hundreds of purveyors of slimming pills, some more convincing than others. Beware the herbal ones — they are often sold in health food shops which somehow seems to give them a respectability and even authenticity. They may have a laxative or diuretic effect; nothing more. Many of them cash in on the grapefruit idea. An idea has been around for centuries that grapefruit is the one substance that actually does burn up fat — another myth, but it has spawned many a grapefruit diet and hundreds of different pills:

The slimmers' natural choice. Unique four-way diet plan. Natural grapefruit extract. Natural fibre and bulking agents. Natural herbal extracts. KLB6.

You pay large sums of money for something that will do you no good and possibly do some harm. KLB6 is meant to sound impressive but is probably phony; even if it is not, no product should contain any substance which is not explained.

THE CAMBRIDGE DIET AND OTHERS

This brings me to the infamous Cambridge Diet and its variations, the UniVite Micro Diet, Herbal Life and a host of others. The Cambridge Diet was developed at Addenbrooke's Hospital, Cambridge and tested there and at the West Middlesex Hospital. Its original purpose was to promote quick weight loss in hospital and under supervision in patients who were considered to be dangerously obese. For several years now it has been available to the public through a local counsellor who advertises in the local press and visits you at home.

The Cambridge Diet and most of its offshoots consist of a sachet of powder to be mixed with water and drunk three times a day. This will give you a daily total of 405 calories. The recommended calorie allowance for a slimming diet for women is usually from 1000-1500 calories daily. So people lose weight very fast on the Cambridge Diet.

> The recent zealous marketing of various formula products to physicians, as well as the public's appetite for such diets could lead to yet another round of complications and fatalities.
>
> The American Medical Association's Council on Scientific Affairs, quoted in NAAFA Newsletter, May 1990

It is monstrous and immoral, exploiting the desire ever-present in women to lose weight and endangering them in the process. It is difficult to know where to start taking this one apart. The leaflet describing the diet — its list of possible minor side effects which do not sound very minor to me — would be enough to make me very suspicious even if I knew nothing about the diet. To embark on something as horrifying as this sounds requires a desperate woman: 'Side effects: headaches, mild dizziness, constipation, diarrhoea, nausea, irritability and dryness of the skin'. The headaches may be the result of dehydration, or caffeine or carbohydrate withdrawal. Constipation could be due to lack of fibre, but you can buy Fybogel for this (oh, and take analgesics for the headaches). The nausea and diarrhoea may be the result of the concentrated minerals and vitamins in the product, or it could be lactose intolerance. Dizziness is the result of the diuretic effect of the diet (I thought this diet was about losing fat, not water). Oh, and you may find you have halitosis (bad breath); use mouthwashes or sprays. Do not drink large quantities of tea or coffee, the caffeine may make you edgy (if you aren't already). And don't drink carbonated, low calorie drinks because they contain sodium which may make the body retain water and slow down the weight loss.

Those are just the minor side effects. Now for the hard facts. VLCDs (very low calorie diets) lower your weight but they also send your metabolism into a state of emergency, signalling to the brain that a famine has begun. So metabolic rate slows down, as it does with any crash diet. This means that last time you lost weight gently on a 1200 calorie a day diet, next time you will have to reduce it to say, 1150 per day to lose the same amount of weight and the more you reduce your metabolic rate the more this figure lowers itself.

When the body is not getting enough calories it does not burn up fat, as people suppose. First it uses the glycogen stored in the liver and then it will make inroads into lean tissue, muscle in other words, and use the protein contained therein as an energy source. Fat people have more lean tissue as well as more fat than thin people and the muscle being eaten into could be vital — the heart muscle for example. Nitrogen in the urine is a sign that lean tissue is being devoured, but there is no way of telling which part of the body that tissue comes from; heart muscle does not identify itself.

Although the Cambridge Diet provides the body with vitamins and minerals, the number of calories ingested is so low as to upset the blood chemistry and blood sugar. There is evidence to suggest that prolonged low blood sugar has an adverse effect on brain cells and will almost certainly cause weakness in someone trying to maintain a normal life-style and do a job. The diuretic effect is also dangerous as that too can upset the blood chemistry.

Taking in so few calories can have the same effect as fasting. The brain produces endorphins which give you a 'high' feeling. Then it can become addictive. I have no statistics for this but I have encountered one case where it happened. A woman was so elated with her weight loss after her month on the Cambridge Diet that she continued with it. After six months she could not stop it, could not resume eating, by which time she had lost more weight than she should have, was dangerously thin, weak and ill. She recovered in the same way that drug addicts do — by weaning herself off her addiction to the diet.

It is unrealistic to remain on 405 calories a day for very long, so what happens when you stop the diet? Inevitably you put on weight, and where you have lost lean tissue and fat, what you will regain will be fat only. When eating is resumed after a VLCD or any kind of crash diet, dangerous stress is put on the cardiovascular system. In one seven-year study in America in which 200 men fasted for a month under medical supervision, 50 of them died in the period following the fast when they started to regain weight, most of them from heart attacks.[19]

The phenomenon I associate with VLCDs is the number of extremely intelligent and sensible women I know who would not dream of doing anything so daft were it not connected with losing weight. As soon as the Grail appears in the mist though, they are chasing it, knowing the risks, knowing too that they will put all that weight back on again. It is as though they are temporarily blinded, can see no further than the shining prospect that in four weeks time they may weigh two stones less, even if in eight weeks time they weigh two and a half stone more.

I know two professional women, close friends, fat all their lives, who made a pact to lose weight together on the Cambridge Diet. When they had lost the weight they threw a party to celebrate (calorie controlled, of course) and gave all their too-big clothes to another (fat) friend of mine. Then I saw them, looking amazingly different, barely recognizable; they had lost *loads* of weight. It made me stop in my tracks for a bit. Surely, I thought, having gone through all that misery and deprivation they will have the incentive to keep the weight off. They did have the incentive, but they reckoned without their bodies. Try as they did, seek desperately for control they might, their bodies threw them into a state of ravenous hunger. They held on for a while, using will-power — anything, everything to keep their new-found figures. Six months later it was all over. They are just a bit fatter than they were before they started the diet. And they have given all their big clothes away to my friend who has benefited enormously and sees no reason to give them back.

One of the most worrying things about VLCDs is that many consultant physicians think they are a *good* treatment for obesity — in fact, the fatter the patient, the more inclined they are to use them. The rationale is that if someone is very fat they are in danger so the weight must be taken off quickly. This does not take into account the fact that the link between obesity *per se* and life-threatening conditions has been found suspect in a number of studies; the fact that VLCDs cause a dangerously quick weight loss which *has* been proven to be life-threatening; nor does it address the problem of maintaining the weight loss — which as any dieter knows, is far less likely to happen if it has been swift.

The Committee on Medical Aspects of Food (COMA) has expressed concern about VLCDs and was instrumental in getting the minimum number of calories raised from 300 to 400 per day (big deal).[20] An article in *The Sunday Times* (London) stated that 'there is a wealth of evidence that, in severe cases of obesity, VLCDs are rapid and effective'. This is nonsense. Even Dr Theodore van Itallie, who is in favour of these liquid diets for the 'very obese' puts the recidivism percentage at anything from 45 to 95, though the lower figure seems unlikely — research shows that 70 per cent of people who use these diets put back the weight lost within one year, and the accepted figure for permanent weight loss is five years. And you cannot keep dieting with a VLCD. However, Van Itallie insists that: 'The liquid diet reduces the psychological burden of dieting (*what! how?*) while controlling nutritional quality. There is always a crisis period after a person has finished the formula diet and has to move back to real food, losing the security of the programme. That is why we offer psychological as well as medical supervision. Any responsible programme has to adopt a multidisciplinary approach with the skills and knowledge to change eating habits and behaviour.'[21] American television personality Oprah Winfrey, with her much publicized Optifast diet, gained back the weight she lost and has vowed never to go on a diet again 'because dieting is the best way of piling on the pounds'.[22]

COMA have also said that VLCDs should be used for no more than three to four weeks at a stretch without medical advice, and their report disagrees with the physicians who prescribe them: 'Very low calorie diets are not generally regarded as a first choice means of achieving weight loss in obese people . . . the use of VLCDs should be considered only after the failure of determined attempts to lose weight with conventional restriction of normal diets . . . very low calorie diets induce a high initial weight loss which can reach over 3kg a week, but this loss includes considerable amounts of fluid and non-fat tissue and is not sustained. Subsequent long-term high rates of weight loss may be at the expense of a disproportionate depletion of non-fat tissues. The effects of weight loss constituted in this way are unknown.' This is a total contradiction of itself. Firstly they say that these diets should only be considered after the failure of ordinary diets (though why the VLCD with its attendant weakness and problems should succeed, I cannot imagine); then they say the weight loss 'is not sustained'.

People have died on very low calorie diets — died while they were still fat. There have been autopsies which have shown *wasted heart muscle* due to lean tissue loss.[23] If all this wasn't scary enough, anyone can get a Cambridge or other diet through untrained salespersons who advertise. I rang my local contact and said I wanted to lose a lot of weight but my doctor didn't approve of the Cambridge diet. Did I need her permission? No, not unless I was on medication, was the answer, and yes, if I wanted to, I could lose weight really fast. The 'counsellor' said that they had brought in a microwave meal that you could have in addition to two liquid replacement meals, but this was only really because the medical profession had been making noises about the full Cambridge diet of three liquid meals (405 calories) per day. You didn't really need the evening meal, she said, and she recommended that I didn't have it if I wanted a quick weight loss. What about these things you read in the papers about quick weight loss being dangerous, I said, and what about this yo-yo dieting? The counsellor did not think either did any harm, but they were always there to help you maintain the weight loss when you finished the diet. Whatever size you are, whatever weight or shape — PLEASE DO NOT TOUCH VERY LOW CALORIE DIETS.

To sum up. Don't put money in the coffers of these manufacturers who are exploiting so many women's most intense desire — to lose weight — so successfully. The only way you can lose weight is by eating a reduced calorie diet and by taking some sort of exercise. But the diet should not be low calorie — 1500-1800 should ensure a slow and steady weight loss and prevent the loss of essential muscle tissue. As for all the rest — if you go into a chemist and feel tempted by expensive meal replacement biscuits, or crunchy 100 calorie sachets, I can only suggest that if your money is burning a hole in your pocket to that extent, then you invest it in shares in one of the well-known and successful companies making these products! While women are addicted to losing weight and gullible enough to believe these wonder claims, your investment can't go wrong.

We lack basic scientific knowledge regarding the causes of obesity. Therefore, our ability to prevent and treat the condition is limited, and the effectiveness of a large number of popular weight-loss and weight-control programs is questionable.

The Surgeon General's Report on Health and Nutrition

SLIMMING CLUBS AND CLINICS

Women do lose weight of course. Many do so through slimming clubs, like Weight Watchers. They work purely through the psychology of group dynamics by shaming or encouraging you to lose weight in the company of others in the same position. The clubs do offer a diet programme but there is nothing special about it. There is nothing special about any carefully worked out diet plan. A slimming diet needs to be high in fibre and unrefined carbohydrates, moderate on protein and low in fat. The only advantage to a programme is that it saves you having to work out the balance, the portions and the calories for yourself.

There is a definite slimming club personality. It is usually competitive and thrives on the congratulations of fellow members as the weight drops off weekly. The slimming club woman enjoys the group discussion where members can relate temptations overcome or succumbed to, triumphs, problems, cooking, family feeding; in short, everything to do with dieting and very little to do with living. It becomes obsessive. The reward-reproach attitude appeals to those who need some form of authority to respond to and to please, who feel shamed when they fail and comforted by the solidarity of others slipping and sliding and climbing up again (or should it be down?).

Bernice Weston says she encouraged Weight Watchers women to become a focal point of the community so that the local mayor would call on them to support charities and so on. While they were doing that, she says, they wouldn't slip back to being fat because it would be letting the side down, and that's a much more powerful motivation than mere self-interest. [24]

But you don't get this for nothing. All slimming clubs have a 'registration fee' and after that you pay for each class. You also pay if you miss a class, however good and genuine your reason. The argument is that paying motivates you to attend; the truth is that it's your money they're after. These are serious business organisations, out to make fat profits like the rest of the industry. Weight Watchers in Britain has 3000 or so branches and in 1992 made a profit of £20 million. It is the most popular of the clubs and many GPs refer their patients — mainly because they do not know how to help people lose weight and they are as confused as the rest of us with all the conflicting information.

I have had two shots at Weight Watchers. Once about 12

years ago, and again in 1992. This last time I survived the diet for under a week but rang my health centre because I was experiencing palpitations, dizziness and breathlessness. I spoke to a health visitor who told me to drop the diet immediately. 'We get a lot of Weight Watchers casualties' she said grimly. I lasted a couple of weeks during my first attempt, and gave it up because I was disgusted and furious to see a completely non-fat, non-overweight child of about twelve being thoroughly chastised by the 'lecturer' because she had lost no weight that week. You might wonder why I went so recently, after speaking out so strongly and publicly against dieting. It was because I am weak and human like everyone else, some of my friends were going, and I thought I would give it a try. Never again. Apart from the fact that I became ill on their diet, I think the whole organization is unethical. Not least in that it encourages young girls to diet. And the age is dropping; about a third of seven-year-old girls would now like to be thinner.[25]

A spokeswoman for Weight Watchers said the company had a very strong policy on young people and only accepted people over the age of ten. This is *monstrous*. The very act of taking a child of that age to a diet club paves the way for a lifetime of problems. It was stated that young people between 10 and 16 must have their family's support and a letter of agreement from their GP.

Every issue of the Weight Watchers magazine features a 'Success of the month'. The November 1992 issue carried the story of a 15-year-old girl, whose mother told Channel 4's *Dispatches*[26] that she had never been asked for a doctor's letter. This is exploitation in the same mould as child pornography.

Nutri/System has been established for a long time in the United States but has only recently arrived in Britain. It's not a club, and it's not exactly a clinic, though the staff wear white coats. It's more of a diet centre, though it runs 'weight loss programmes' rather than diets. Prospective clients fill in a detailed questionnaire which is sent to their GP. They have a counselling session and buy prepared, packaged food. The appeal of this method is supposed to lie in the reassuring 'counsellors' (who may have had absolutely no medical or nutritional training before joining the staff), and in the 'safety' of foods prepared and ready to eat, planned and calorie counted, rather like the Weight Watchers range of meals.

Mike Householder was 44, and Dean of Engineering at a university. He wanted to lose 30lb and went to Nutri/System. He took away the prepacked food, followed the diet — 1000 calories per day — and exercised, jogging for 30 minutes a day. He lost the 30lb in two months — over 3lb per week. He was tired and weak — and one day he fainted. He told the staff at the centre. They suggested he added a little more fruit to his diet. He did so, but soon after he had a cardiac arrest. He was in a coma for three days and when he came round he had no memory at all. He didn't know who he was, didn't recognize his wife and children, remembered nothing of his life before the cardiac arrest. His memory has not fully returned and he is no longer capable of doing his job. Now he and his wife run a guesthouse. The family are loving and have stayed together but Carol Householder still weeps when she talks about what happened. He's changed, she says.

Nutri/System claimed there was no connection between Mike's cardiac arrest and their diet. However, for a man of his age who is jogging 30 minutes a day, 1000 calories is dangerously inadequate. His cardiologist found that Mike was short of potassium — this can happen on an insufficient calorie intake, especially when combined with fluid loss through exercise. He was also found to have existing coronary heart disease. The physician feels the diet had some part to play in his cardiac arrest. Nutri/System made a large financial settlement out of court, enabling Mike and Carol to buy the guesthouse. Seven years on, he has had no recurrent cardiac trouble, which his doctor feels is another indication that the diet was implicated in the cardiac arrest. If medical supervision were adequate, why did the diet centre ignore the warning signs — weakness, tiredness and fainting?

Rapid weight loss diets with insufficient calories are now thought to be linked with gallstones and gallbladder disease. There has been a spate of Nutri/System clients with gallbladder disease who have brought lawsuits against the company. Many clients have been paid out of court.

The United States is ahead of Britain in its investigations of the diet industry. Several products have been taken off the market. Diet centres are checked out. The New York City Department of Consumer Affairs produced a report: 'A Weighty Issue: Dangers and Deceptions of the Weight Loss Industry' after staff members posed as dieters at 14 New York centres or clinics, including Nutri/System, Optifast, Medifast and the Slim Time Weight Loss Center. A Department of Consumer Affairs Commissioner concluded that 'To these centers, a pound of fat is worth a pound of profit — all too often at the expense of the dieter's health and well-being.' The report proposed, among other conditions, that diet centres should 'affirmatively disclose in advertisements and oral presentations that there are serious health risks associated with rapid weight loss, and that rapid weight loss has not been proven effective on a long-term basis'.[27]

The American National Institute of Health has stated its intention to put the physical and psychological cosequences of dieting right at the top of the health agenda. Four congressional hearings were held, all of which were critical of the diet industry. Congressman Ron Wyden said that American consumers were spending over $30 billion a year on weight loss programmes and products. All too often the results were poor and occasionally even life-threatening.

The British government appears to be doing now what the American National Institute of Health did in 1985 when the Consensus Development Conference on the Health Implications of Obesity pronounced it a 'killer disease', without taking account of the harmful effects of dieting and the immense power of the industry. Now there is a Government white paper — 'The Health of the Nation' — which aims for a 40 per cent reduction in premature deaths from heart disease by encouraging a large proportion of the population to lose weight. There is no mention of the hazards of dieting itself.

There is a strong tide of feeling on both sides of the Atlantic that the power and profit of the diet industry *must* be curtailed. The Advertising Standards Association and the Trading Board in Britain need to be much more active in consumer protection. The government has left it to the market, but it has been a market which has capitalised on public clamour for anything that will make them magically lose weight. In the business of slimming, objective judgement goes out of the window and the diet industry has taken full advantage of this. As one woman said: 'I've tried every new gimmick that's come on the market, and I know I'll keep trying. The lure of the miracle cure is impossible to resist. You'll spend anything if you want to lose weight and they know it, so they've got a ready made fortune — every day. It's a great, big con.'

However, there is a far more serious kind of exploitation going on and one where the law cannot act. These are the slimming clinics, which you can find advertised in women's magazines and local newspapers and magazines. I looked in one London magazine and found several offering a three- or four-week course of medication for between £50 and £60. I rang them all for details and was told I would be given pills to help suppress my appetite. One said they had six different kinds of appetite suppressants and that one woman lost thirteen pounds in her first week. They all reassured me that I didn't have to have my doctor's permission and the clinics themselves would not get in touch with my doctor if I did not wish them to. These appetite suppressants are, of course, a dangerous group of highly addictive drugs, the amphetamines, or speed. They are powerful, only obtainable on prescription and have serious side-effects, including depression and hallucinations, and they come under the control of the Misuse of Drugs Act 1971.

In an edition of the BBC chat show, *Kilroy*, women talked of the effects slimming pills had had on them:

> I changed personality — I tried to kill my husband with a carving knife — I couldn't stop myself.

> You feel as if you're snapping — you go up and down. It damaged my health. I wanted to keep nice and slim and sexy.

> I lost my memory completely.

> My personality changed completely — I was impulse buying, I had insomnia, itching, palpitations, hot flushes, shaking.[28]

The Pharmaceutical Society of Great Britain is powerless even though it has received many complaints. The law permits the handing out of these drugs even though there may be no doctor on the clinic premises.

In March 1988, the *Observer* published a report after sending three human guinea pigs to a slimming clinic.[29] None of them was overweight to any degree; they could in fact have been anorexic. But one woman, Annabel Ferriman, who at 5′ weighed 7st. 4lb (105lb) was given the weight of 6st. 13lb (97lb) for the lower end of her 'ideal' range.

The doctor in charge of the clinic was evasive. When asked why the women had not been checked for pregnancy his reply was that 'Pregnant women do not come to slimming clinics. People are not that dumb'. The *Observer* reporter questioned him about the prescribing of drugs for people as slim as Annabel Ferriman. He replied that women were strange and that there were people who were just as slim as Annabel who wanted to lose weight. And there, of course, he is right. But Dr John Garrow, Professor of Human Nutrition at St Bartholomew's Hospital said he would not use these drugs on even the most obese person.

The only action the law allows is the prosecution of these clinics for supplying unlabelled drugs. The Pharmaceutical Society has secured several such convictions with fines as low as £250. Apart from the risk to health there is a very real danger. The amphetamine-like substances cause irregular heart rhythms, as can the diuretics which unbalance the blood chemistry.

Since the law offers no protection and magazines continue to carry advertisements for these clinics, it is essential that no woman ever buys any kind of pill to aid slimming. At best they will be placebos. At worst they carry a severe risk.

You may have heard about the talking scales that reprimand you bossily if you put on an ounce, and the electronic device on the fridge door that whines at you not to stuff yourself again because you're turning into a fat pig. Dozens of gadgets like these are available.

For those who really fear they may lose control, there are the Diet Cops. Carrie Latt Wiatt runs Diet Designs in Los Angeles where it caters for a rich and influential clientele. Carrie trains her clients to eat properly; she 'feels about butter the way Greenpeace feels about nuclear waste'. She visits people's kitchens, clearing fridges of offending foods, sometimes reducing her clients to tears with her hard-line approach. 'I'm part diet shrink, part Hitler' she says of herself, and replaces what she considers junk with her own foods. The first consultation costs $150, during which Ms Latt Wiatt takes a thorough medical, dietary and lifestyle history. After that, the weekly fee is $200 and you receive diet instructions and a paper bag containing your first three days' food.

If clients are going to eat out, Ms Latt Wiatt telephones the restaurant informing them of her clients' arrival and saying what they may or may not be served. Having provided food for five days a week, this tough woman will teach them (or their chefs) how to prepare and cook her meals. This service costs $750.[30] It's really a grown up version of a stern 'Mother-knows-best' approach and clients seem to love it.

There are some bizarre and totally useless products promising a new slim you. You can try an electronic pulse slimming belt, rather like the Slendertone type of treatment. Or sweat-it-out sauna suits. I hope no-one is silly enough to buy them. Even so, they do not have the ruthless, exploitative profit motive of the mainline industry and they will only harm your pocket, not your health. They are eccentrically useless, but no more so than exercise videos, for example, some of which can be risky as they demand too much from bodies which may not be up to it. But there will always be crazes — like step aerobics, for which you are supposed to buy expensive equipment when you probably have a perfectly good flight of stairs in your own home.

There are a number of creams, lotions and gels, mudpacks and seaweed baths which claim to break down, or firm up your flab. Costing up to about £50 a jar or pot, the only thing they will lighten will be your bank balance. These potions work through the skin as a diuretic, or encourage circulation by dilating the capillaries on the skin surface; or they may temporarily tighten the skin itself. What they cannot do is to shift the fat beneath the skin. The eternally boring cellulite debate which produces all sorts of electrical and chemical treatments at inflated prices to deflate thighs does not remove fat either. Cellulite — the hard, lumpy tissue which so many women are practically suicidal about and which usually forms on thighs — is best removed, if it exists at all, by increasing the circulation of both the blood and lymphatic systems: by simple exercise, free walks or cycle rides, or perhaps the price of the entrance fee to your local swimming bath. If you have money that you wish to spend on being kind to your body, then spend it on massage. You won't lose weight, but you will feel invigorated and relaxed and purring all over. It's a delicious experience and one that should be sought for pure pleasure, not in the cause of self-improvement.

SURGERY, OR SELF-MUTILATION

I realise that I have just committed blasphemy in the eyes of the 80 per cent or so who would like to lose weight, or change shape. Self-indulgence of the body is what causes all our problems, remember? Jane Walmsley, whose ideal weight at 5'4", is an anorexic seven and a half stones (105lbs), wrote an article called 'The Unprincipled Body' (what else could it be called?) advocating drastic and stern measures to fight our flab. In this smug piece of propaganda — having attained her magical weight she resolved to follow a diet for ever and has done so — Walmsley says she has little patience with the 'infirm of purpose'. As for 'Size 16 and beautiful — coming to terms with your weight', Ms Walmsley calls that a cop-out, 'Like writing an article called "How to stop worrying and love the bomb".' Ms Walmsley's imagery is so violent in fact that it is clear that she has a problem with her body in spite of her mockery of the beautiful size 16s. Anyone who can take a (sinful, of course) bite out of a blueberry muffin, throw it in the waste bin, retrieve it covered in cigarette ash and *then* eat it, has no more found peace with the world or her body than unhappy fat people.

There is only one way to discipline the body, she says: 'If you want them (fat cells) to move, you've got to bludgeon them to death.' And a paragraph later: 'Female fat is the stubbornest stuff since Arthur Scargill, and you can't get rid of it unless you club it to death over extended periods'.[31]

Clubbing flesh to death has never been so popular, nor have ways to do it been so available to women until recently. No longer do they have to rely on dieting to kill their bodies; there are other means at their disposal, at a price — not only the price they pay in money. The following account reads like one of those hospital horror stories where surgery has either been very major or gone horribly wrong:

> *Day one*
> I come round from the anaesthetic shaking violently. Every muscle of my thighs feels like a rubber band being pulled out in different directions. I wish I had been warned about this. I am hooked from the waist to below the knees in an unbelievably unglamorous corset.
> *Day two*
> The pain is awful. I can go home.
> *Day three*
> A rotten night, much pain. Needed strong painkiller. Feet and ankles very swollen.
> *Day five*
> Shopping. I feel very odd and I have to sit down. When I get home I find that even my knees are swelling round the end of the corset.

Day six

I am sleeping badly and decide that a painkiller every night is not a sign of weakness.

Day eight

To Harley Street for the removal of the stitches. As the corset is peeled off I gasp with horror. The insides and outsides of both thighs are BLACK. My knees are very swollen and my thighs feel solid. The surgeon seems quite pleased. He tells me to massage each of them for ten minutes each night and morning to get the circulation going and dispose of the lumps.

Day nine

I have been told to walk a lot and not to stand still but for me this is impossible; I have very swollen legs at the end of the day so am giving them a double massage. Before I finish, I will have kneaded five big jars of cold cream into the horrible thick lumps which have to be broken up on the inside of each thigh. I still hate struggling into that wretched corset.

Day eighteen

I still have a huge lump on the inside of my right thigh and several knobbly ones on the left. The blackness has broken up into distinguishable bruises, undulating like threatening thunderclouds on a particularly nasty summer's day. But to my joy I can already see that I look a lot better in slacks and straight skirts.

Day thirty-one

All the swelling has at last gone and ninety per cent of the soreness and I've lost four inches round the thigh area and two around each knee.

Six months later

The surgeon noticed a slight unevenness. Therefore he extracted, free of charge, a little more fat from a small bulge. Now the thighs are completely even and I have got what I hoped for — a much slimmer line . . . and I am even going out to buy a pair of shorts.[32]

The woman who wrote the above account was not having a major therapeutic operation. She was undergoing liposuction, now the most popular cosmetic operation in the United States and becoming increasingly so over here. She was satisfied with the top half of her body, due to frequent dieting and was not overweight, but felt self-conscious when her legs were revealed.

This form of mutilation involves converting the fat into a liquefied form and inserting several long metal tubes into the skin. These cannulae are attached to a pump; when it is switched on the fat is sucked out as yellow sludge into a calibrated glass container. It is considered unwise to remove more than two kilograms at any one time. I have not seen liposuction performed but the description of the suction pump and cannulae reminds me of the time I saw a dead body embalmed; then, blood and organic matter was sucked out via a cannula and pump and deposited into a glass container.

An ideal patient presenting herself for liposuction of the breasts was Karen, a tall, slim blonde who weighed nine stones and did not like her large breasts. She did not find it easy to wear a bikini. The surgeon separated her nipples with what he called a 'cookie cutter' then resited them, having first used liposuction to sculpt and remove the fat on her breasts. The nipples ended up three inches higher so that she would have nice small high breasts and the skin was tightened. Now she was a perfect woman.

Liposuction on various parts of the body costs from £2000–4000, and a great deal of pain, swelling and scarring if any knifework is performed as well. Breast reduction or mammoplasty is a demolition and rebuild job. Much of the breast tissue is removed and what remains is reshaped into an 'acceptable' compact, round, smaller breast. The nipples have to be detached and resited, which results in loss of sensation and it will not be possible to breastfeed a baby.

This particular surgery is fraught with potentially serious complications — breasts may retain hard lumps of tissue and blood clots can occur. Some years ago I mentioned to a doctor friend that I was considering breast reduction and asked her how to go about it. 'Don't' she said baldly. She had heard that week that a patient of hers, about my age and thinner, who had gone for the surgery had died from an embolus — a blood clot lodged in the heart or lungs. And for this pain, discomfort and risk of death you can expect to pay around £3000–£5000.

Having dealt with breasts and thighs, not to mention the odd liposuction session on arms, face, or wherever, what about our vast stomachs? Well, we could have abdominoplasty for around £4000, known as the tummy tuck. This is for the Big Sag, usually caused by pregnancy, where muscles and skin are stretched. It can also occur in middle age where fat tends to be laid down on the abdominal wall; the middle-age spread we call it. Excess skin and fat are removed and bellies are flattened by tightening the abdominal muscles with thick permanent sutures. This is described as a debilitating major operation, but think of the lovely flat bikini stomach after all the pain has gone.

For the removal of fat over the entire abdominal area, as opposed to tightening the sag, you will need an apronectomy. You will have two large incisions, one horizontal, one vertical, 'so that the woman looks like a hot cross bun' as one surgeon described it to me so pictorially. Fat will be cut out and the incisions sewn up. Again this is a major operation, with a high price tag.

If the descriptions haven't put you off and you have that sort of money lying around in the bank, just wait before you rush off to book yourself any of these. The ultimate in ironies is that these operations are not available to fat people. They are for stubborn areas of fat on thighs or hips, or for the sag caused by pregnancy, or yo-yo dieting, or age. A cosmetic surgeon will require you to lose weight if you are more than a very little overweight. And once you've had the operation you must not put weight back on again. So it would appear that it's all back to dieting again.

So why are these operations available and why are they so popular? They are not for 'real people'. The tall slim blonde, Karen, who underwent the liposuction and reconstruction of her breasts to make them small and high so that she could wear a bikini again; the diary of the woman who endured such pain in order to have 'perfect' thighs; the young woman I met who had just one pound of fat removed from her upper thighs in order to become perfect, and who fainted from the pain when the anaesthetic wore off — they all reminded me of the film *The Stepford Wives* in which normal, gutsy women were turned into perfect flawless robots by their collaborating husbands. But that is what it is all about.

I talked to one Australian cosmetic surgeon now practising in this country and he informed me that these operations were far more common in Australia. This man spoke of his work as 'creating perfection' and the word perfection occurred frequently in his descriptions of the operations he performed. He explained that they were almost routine in Australia because men demanded a greater degree of 'perfection' from their women, were more macho in their refusal to allow their women to let themselves go. Did he think that this was less prevalent in Britain because the men were more tolerant, their standards of perfection somewhat less demanding? No way, he said. It was because British men were *wimps* and they allowed their women to let themselves go far too much.

If in spite of everything you cannot resist the idea of a fat-reducing cosmetic operation, be very careful where you go to obtain it. You will find them advertised in plenty of magazines, but it is important that you keep to the forefront

The Barbie doll is the ultimate symbol of our oppression, the bane of our existence! It has long been my conviction that those who would keep women in their places invented a doll which embodied the look of their 'ideal woman' . . . She was tall, extremely thin, with body proportions that occur extremely rarely in actual women's bodies, with thighs that never rub together, 'big' hair, feet deformed from constantly wearing high-heeled shoes, and outfits and accessories that glorify and promote self-absorption, primping, exhibitionism, and materialistic behaviour.

Lynn Meletiche, NAAFA Newsletter, December 1992

'Ever since I was a little girl I wanted to look like a Barbie doll' says Cindy Jackson. 'She doesn't have moles or wrinkles — I mean *look* at her skin.' Cindy, a 28-year-old rock singer, gave up her flat and sold her family jewellery to pay for surgery. Her new 'Barbie' body cost her £20,400 (it would cost considerably more now). Cindy said: 'I was a bimbo trapped inside a hill-billy body and face.' Addiction to cosmetic surgery is now a recognised psychiatric condition.

Daily Mail, 27 May 1991

Many cosmetic surgeons perform numerous operations on their wives with the idea of making them perfect. One surgeon, referring to the annual dinner dance for Plastic and Reconstructive surgeons said the same wives 'look better every year . . . One surgeon so completely rearranged his wife that we didn't recognise her. She was a walking advertisement'.

From *Allure*, April 1992

of your mind that these people are in this business to make money. It is not the same as cosmetic reconstruction after an accident or as a result of a congenital deformity. This is going with the wave of media dictatorship and providing the answer for women who are so deeply influenced by it.

There are reputable professional organizations acting as watchdogs on the cosmetic surgery industry, like the British Association of Aesthetic Plastic Surgeons who have stated that although not all commercial clinics are dubious, there are only two or three really reputable ones in the country. If you answer an advertisement you risk being treated by a surgeon who is simply not competent to perform your operation. It is best to check by contacting either the Medical Advisory Service or the Harley Street Medical Advisory Service.[33]

Apart from the cosmetic business, which makes millions of pounds out of women's vanity — and before I am attacked for that remark, isn't it vanity to pay several hundred pounds to have a pound of flesh removed from your thighs? — there are the weight-loss operations, some of which were invented in the USA and all performed there, and here on the NHS, by doctors who consider drastic treatment is necessary for obesity.

The two simplest, the wearing of an unremovable nylon cord around the waist and jaw-wiring, seem to me to be the most humiliating. Maybe it is my Catholic background but I am frequently reminded when discussing or writing about the things women do to kill their flesh of the Catholic practice of mortifying the flesh. And to mortify actually means to kill; used in this context, to bring the flesh into subjection, to discipline. The discipline of a nylon cord round your waist, its ends fused together means that if you eat more than moderately the cord cuts in and if you put on any weight it can be agony. Its inventor was a man who does not seem to have taken into consideration the fluctuations in weight and girth caused by women's hormones and water retention, so truly it seems a punishing device. Nevertheless it has to be said that it is the women who agree to wear it.

Jaw-wiring is even more humiliating and frightening and dangerous. The teeth are wired together so that the victim cannot open her mouth to talk or eat. She can drink some form of liquid diet. This does not appear to be at all effective. Many women lose a great deal of weight, but as jaw-wiring does not tackle the cause of the weight gain, the weight usually returns when the wires are removed. And temptation is still there: you can consume a large number of calories in a liquid or blended form. When your jaws are wired together you cannot speak except through gritted teeth, literally. And there is always the danger of vomiting and choking on it because of the force behind it and the lack of an exit. It is so ineffectual it seems nothing more than a form of discipline or punishment for the condition of fatness — hardly the cure, or even a therapy.

The most effective surgical procedure for the reduction of weight is the intestinal bypass developed in the 1960s. This reduces the normal length of the intestines from about twenty feet to about one foot. Food cannot be digested or absorbed, leading to severe diarrhoea and malnutrition, and patients quickly learn to eat less to avoid digestive upsets. However it has been found that even the short length of intestine left to the patient can adapt to some extent and gradually becomes thicker and longer, improving its ability to extract nutrients from food. This is often accompanied by weight gain, though it is slow. There have been a considerable number of fatalities with the bypass operation and for this reason it was discontinued; however it is beginning to make a come-back due to research which has led to improved techniques.

It is performed more frequently in America than in

Britain, and in spite of the high risk and the dangerous after-effects it is considered justifiable as an emergency measure in the case of morbid obesity. The imponderable is the definition of morbid obesity. There are many more very fat people in America than in Britain — I am talking about people weighing thirty to forty stones (400--600 lb) or more; there are Americans (men) weighing 73 and 86 stones (1000 and 1200 lb).[34] They cannot move even to get out of bed and it is obvious that they are in need of a life-saving procedure. But they are exceptional and the life-threatening risks of this surgery itself must be taken into consideration. One after-effect is liver damage leading to liver failure and death and a total of thirty-seven complications arising from this operation have been documented. One estimate of the risk is that someone undergoing this surgery is about nine times more likely to die than someone of the same age, weight and sex who has not had surgery.[35]

The most popular method of surgical weight loss is the stomach stapling operation though there are in fact about two dozen variations of this. The stomach is made much smaller with a surgical staple gun, reducing its capacity from the normal quart or so down to about two ounces. The patient is forced on to the equivalent of a crash diet and rapidly loses weight. This operation is no magic solution though; the stomach adapts and has an almost infinite capacity for stretching. The only way stomach stapling is effective in the long term is by careful maintenance of diet, so it would seem easier and safer to diet in the first place, and by a safer method than the crash diet. The American Medical Association has produced figures estimating that 2 to 4 per cent of patients undergoing stomach stapling die within a few days of surgery. The death rate may be higher due to potentially fatal complications that can crop up later, including irregular heartbeat, brain and nerve damage, stomach cancer, immune deficiency, pernicious anaemia and liver failure.

At Manchester Royal Infirmary in Britain the operation is used only on patients with what is termed 'morbid obesity'. This unfortunate term is in itself contentious as 'experts' vary in their definition of it. Vincent Taylor, a surgeon at M.R.I., has described the operation as 'a method of physical restraint ... major surgery. We staple the stomach to create a small pouch holding only 20 cubic centimetres, and put a silicone band round the outlet of the pouch to slow down the rate of emptying'. As well-known writer and broadcaster Libby Purves commented: 'In other words the patient is left with a stomach the length of a pen and the prospect of an invalidish diet for life.'[36]

Annette Connolly, who talked about the operation on a gruesome edition of the BBC documentary *40 Minutes*[37] can no longer digest red meat, oranges, bananas or apples. She said 'I feel a bit like Frankenstein's monster, as if I've been mutilated.' Annette was 16 stones (224lb) before the operation and had diabetes. At the time of the documentary, she was around 10½ stones and sticking to her diet — not that gastroplasty patients have much choice.

This operation is, I believe, open to a number of ethical questions. In the United States, for example, it is often done for what could be termed cosmetic rather than medical reasons; and has been offered as a solution to women of much lower weights — 10-11 stones (140-154 lb). It also appears that the reasons for performing it are often not examined adequately, if at all. Annette Connelly had diabetes, was fat, was told this was a risk and so had the operation. Kath O'Donnell, who appeared on the same programme, was just fat. She said: 'I was fat because I ate for comfort and when I couldn't do that any more, I panicked. I couldn't cope with my life without the food. I ate and ate and ruined everything.' The staples in her stomach burst open. She tried the operation again and *within a year* she went from 19 stones to 7 (265-98 lb) and got dangerously dehydrated. The band was taken off, and her weight went up again, then she got an ulcer. At the time of the programme she had undergone her *fourth* gastroplasty operation. 'If I don't get it right this time, there's no hope.'

When I reached 20 stones (280 lb) I had my jaw wired. It worked and I got down to 10 stones (140 lb). I felt really good about myself but within two years my weight had shot up to 18 stones (252 lb) and I went on the Cambridge Diet. That worked too, and I stopped it when I reached 12 stones (168 lb) thinking that with a sensible diet I could continue to lose weight. I did eat carefully but stopping the Cambridge Diet sent my weight rocketing again, this time to 19 stones (266 lb). I went to ask about stomach-stapling and was told I could have it if I got down to 14 stones (196 lb). I had my jaw wired yet again to help me and have just reached the required weight. The operation is booked but I have suddenly realised what I have been doing to myself. I am going to cancel the operation, eat sensibly and just see what my weight does. I can't believe that I've subjected myself to such violence.

I had my teeth wired together several years ago so that I could lose a lot of weight. I didn't realise that the dentist would grind them all down and the pain was incredible. I was terrified of choking, even though I had to carry a pair of wire-cutters everywhere just in case. The weight came off though because I could only take liquids. As soon as the wires were removed I started to put the weight back on. So I had my stomach stapled. No one told me about the pain, the heartburn and the vomiting. Sometimes I feel convinced that I'm having a heart attack. I wish I hadn't done it.

From personal letters to the author.

These women suffered from the low esteem of the fat woman but did not see the problem as a result of society's persecution. They were women with no idea of the meaning of consciousness-raising. They had had no counselling or therapy, so they put themselves in the hands of the medical profession, whose answer was to put them under the knife and the staple-gun. 'He is lovely, Mr Taylor,' they said of the surgeon. 'But it is a horrible operation.' Kath O'Donnell now realizes that she needs counselling.

Women who have undergone gastroplasty report a number of effects, some unpleasant, some distressing, some truly terrifying. They range from the discomfort when they eat even a tiny amount more than the stomach's capacity (though the effect of this is to stretch the stomach, which makes the surgery self-defeating) through to the most extreme pain; one woman spoke of the necessity to chew everything into pulp, otherwise she would vomit. The act of vomiting itself was agony and caused her such severe chest pain she kept thinking she must be having a heart attack. Another reported 'successful' weight loss, but said that the symptoms associated with the operation were growing worse all the time. These included severe pain in the whole of her digestive tract and excessive stomach acid causing almost continuous heartburn. Others talk about the frightening symptoms of the rapid weight loss itself: the dizziness, palpitations, and weakness. There is malnutrition because the body is not taking enough calories, vitamins and minerals and supplements are necessary. The necessity to chew everything so finely means that it is tempting to eat soft, creamy foods like chocolate mousse or ice cream. The point about this operation is that although your food intake is physically controlled, you are still on a permanent diet, watching *what* you eat, and how much. If you binge in desperation, the consequences are horrendous, as Kath O'Donnell found. If you just eat gradual but ever-increasing amounts, the stomach capacity expands and you can end up weighing as much as before the operation.

Another method involves inserting a balloon in your stomach via a tube through which the balloon is then inflated with something like a bicycle pump. The idea is that you feel full but, again, careful attention must be paid to what the doctors call 'dietary discipline'. The balloon which was invented in America was designed for people at least 100 per cent over their recommended weight. The American Food and Drug Administration ignored this cautious estimate from the inventor himself and approved the balloon for virtually anyone. The balloon is said to be safer than bypass or stapling but it too has risks, the greatest being that it may deflate and lodge in the intestine. It has caused some fatalities. It is really only an incentive to weight loss by diet because it cannot be kept permanently in the stomach.

Immediately after the death of Christina Onassis in October 1988, amidst speculation that her death was caused by slimming pills, the BBC ran an edition of its audience participation programme, *Kilroy*, on the subject of aids to weight loss. Grimly entitled 'Dying For your Figure', the programme featured women who had tried everything from amphetamines to all forms of surgical intervention. The 'success story' was Shirley, who was gaunt and ill-looking, greyish-pale and haggard. She had had an intestinal bypass ten years earlier when she weighed twenty-four and a half stones (345 lb). Following her rapid weight loss she had then undergone a number of cosmetic operations. 'I looked like a deflated balloon,' she said. 'I sagged everywhere'. Shirley had reductions done on her stomach, her legs and her bust. She then had her bust *enlarged* with silicon implants. She doesn't regret it, she feels she had no choice as she had been told she would not live much longer at the weight she was.

That is where things go wrong. She knew she was taking a risk with the bypass operation. She was warned that there had been deaths. She had to undergo a considerable amount of pain and risk with the additional cosmetic operations. The world's largest epidemiological study followed 1.8 million participants for ten years. The typical weight-loss surgery patient is a woman in her thirties who is 100 pounds overweight by the charts. She can expect to live another forty years. She could add a maximum of five years to her life expectancy by losing weight, but only if she can maintain that loss . . . and achieve it safely. Any method that is potentially dangerous or that cannot ensure permanent weight reduction will shorten, not lengthen that woman's life expectancy.[38] It is essential that before embarking on any weight-loss procedure there is complete certainty that the benefits will outweigh the risks.

Another woman on *Kilroy* described how she had reduced from thirty-one stones (435lb) to eleven (154lb) with stomach stapling. She seemed fit and in fact was pregnant. But she was only able to eat a quarter of a Weetabix for breakfast, half an egg for lunch and what she called a 'small cocktail' for tea. No nutritionist would give approval to that as a diet for a pregnant woman.

A young woman, in my opinion and that of several people who watched the programme with me, the most attractive and healthy looking on the show, said she had received a gastric balloon at Addenbrookes Hospital in Cambridge. Her stomach tried to reject it and she said for three days she did not know whether she was going to die, the pain was such she thought she was having a heart attack. In spite of that, and with the balloon removed, she said she would do anything to stop being fat, consider any other measure however drastic. She said she had tried to commit suicide because she could not face living with the pressure of being stigmatised. This young woman was glowingly beautiful.

Richard Harrison, a surgeon who had carried out many stapling operations, said of the procedure that this operation does not remove the need to diet. He was answering the query of a woman who said that after the operation she could only eat teaspoonfuls, but now she could take much more. It all comes back to diet.

But women do see both the cosmetic and the surgical operations as the instant answer and it is easy to see how this could be. It sounds wonderful — a short, easy route to a slim body and no more worries about health, or nagging by doctors, or social ostracism. But the risks must be considered and these operations regarded as dangerous and certainly not to be undergone for the sake of vanity. In America the National Association to Advance Fat Acceptance has issued a statement strongly criticizing present surgical approaches to weight loss. And there is an increase in the number of malpractice suits being filed against surgeons.

Researchers and doctors like Paul Ernsberger and Paul Haskew have consistently warned of the risk of surgical procedures for weight loss. Sixty possible complications and risks have been found. And we know that dieting does not work. So what is the fat woman to do if she wants to be healthy? Can you, in fact, be fat and fit, despite a lifetime of being told you cannot?[39]

7

So you think you're fat: the health facts and figures

Going into the medical picture of obesity is like stepping into a minefield. You have to accept that no one really knows to what extent being fat endangers health because so many other factors have to be considered. There is no definite answer, but within the medical profession there are a multitude of theories ranging from those that completely oppose each other to those that agree, with some degree of overlap.

The most recent official medical report in Britain is that of the Royal College of Physicians in 1983. It starts by giving tables based on those used by life insurance companies, showing what we should weigh according to height. Looking at the tables I see that the 'acceptable average' for me is 8st. 1 lb (113lb), though at the lower end of the range I could be expected to weigh as little as 7st. 4lb (102lb). This does not explain why I felt so fit at 12 stones (168lb); nor why I have been told by more than one doctor, during my dieting days, that it would not be healthy for me to weigh less than 10 stones (140lb). Looking further at the chart I learn that my daughter — a beautiful girl, perfectly proportioned at 5'5" with long slender legs, slim waist, well-formed breasts and flat stomach — is to be considered overweight. She should weigh, at the lower end of the range for her height, 7st. 13lb (111lb); her 'acceptable average' is 8st. 11lb (123lb). At 9st. 5lb (131lb) she had better watch out, according to these charts; though she does not exceed the upper limit, it is only a matter of a few pounds before she does so. My husband was chastised at a medical examination for being at the upper end of the 'normal' weight range! He was advised to aim for the lower band of 'normal' even though his build is medium to heavy.

I do not propose to discuss anorexia in this book for several reasons: it has been written about to saturation point, and the anorexic girl or woman is the object of social sympathy mixed with a certain amount of admiration. Self-destructive she may be, but the anorexic has visibly demonstrated self-discipline and self-control which people cannot help admiring. Nonetheless it is an illness which is escalating each year; it *is* a worry for the mothers of teenage girls. It has been known as 'the Slimmers' Disease' and looking at these weight charts and then at my beautiful, slim daughter I can see why she is already beginning to be troubled by her weight. And I am very angry at the pressure she is under, and find the preoccupation with thinness equalling perfection an understandable response in teenage girls, most of whom have not yet developed sufficient sense of personal identity to be different from the crowd in any way.

Out of interest, I checked on the weights of several people who are slim, as opposed to bonily thin. Maureen, a college PE instructor, fast and fit with a tiny waist, came out at half a stone overweight for the chart. The only people — and it was mainly women I was looking at — who satisfied the requirements of this weight chart were those who are truly thin, not slim, whose bones stick out, who have hollows and 'salt cellars' where there is no flesh to sit comfortably between the bones and who are flat-chested and bemoan the fact. In fact, the women with a basically androgynous figure. Those women, whom nobody would call fat but who weighed perhaps two stones above the tables' acceptable weight range, are medically defined as 'obese' as opposed to overweight which means exceeding the limit by not very much. The report goes on to say bleakly that this may well carry a risk of early death. Having said that, the report does go on to cite some studies which have shown that the lowest mortality rate exists among middle-aged people who are overweight (in the medical sense) or 'mildly obese'. And it does admit to the greater hazards to health and life expectancy associated with smoking. The weight gain which may follow when someone stops smoking is considered less risky than remaining a smoker.

To sum up: the report pulls no punches in its descriptions of the risk of increased incidence of diabetes, gall-bladder disease, hypertension, arthritis, respiratory problems and cancer in fat women and men. Most overweight people, though, are usually warned, by their doctors as well as everyone else (people are inclined to claim the right to speak to fat people as though they were subnormal or not entitled to the usual social courtesy and respect), that it is their heart that is really at risk, and it is that, with its immediate life-threatening danger, which frightens and intimidates the overweight patient in the doctor's consulting room. While stating clearly and sternly that obesity does indeed lead to a substantially increased risk of angina and sudden death, not to put too fine a point on it, the report does allow that overweight is considered to be a less important risk factor than age, sex, hypertension, smoking and raised blood fats (hyperlipidaemia). Indeed one report is cited[1] which demonstrates that the Africans living in South Africa have a high prevalance of obesity *without* the associated morbidity and mortality. The reasons given for this are environmental — factors such as diet. The most significant difference here is that though clinically described as obese, the Africans have a diet very low in fat and high in fibre-rich unrefined carbohydrates; quite different from the Western diet of the affluent societies which is high in fat. It is now agreed almost unanimously in the medical profession that a high fat diet leads to high blood fats, leading in turn to Coronary Heart Disease (CHD).

Ancel Keys postulates that the cross-cultural[2] differences in CHD show that obesity should not be used as a causal factor.

Paul Ernsberger tried to find the link between overweight and blood pressure using white rats.[3] He gave one group the normal Purina Rat Chow and the other group were fed on high-calorie foods. They developed twice the amount of baby fat as the other rats but their heart function and blood pressure remained normal. Fat animals eat the same number of calories each day and their weight remains stable; a far cry, says Ernsberger, from the existence of most fat people who diet and starve and yo-yo up and down the scale.

To mimic this situation, the rats were put on a partial fast for four days (something like our Cambridge Diet). Their blood pressure dropped, and stabilised, falling no further after the second day though the rats continued to lose weight. In dieting humans, a similar pattern of blood pressure has been found.[4] Within two days of the end of their 'crash diet' the rats' blood pressure had shot up to its previous level, though at that stage they had regained only a fraction of the weight they had lost. As the human dieter regains weight after a rapid loss, the lowered blood pressure rises and reaches a higher level than at the start of the diet. Ernsberger's rats went through four cycles imitating human dieting and regaining weight, and at the end of this they appeared to have developed permanently high blood pressure.

Yo-yo dieting also affects blood pressure and heart function through the release of a stress hormone, noradrenalin, through the nervous system. Noradrenalin itself actually damages the walls of the arteries which then have to be repaired by a clotting substance, fibrinogen. The more repairs that are needed, the more our arteries become clogged with fibrinogen.[5] Noradrenalin is also released under emotional stress so it will affect us when we are insulted, stigmatised, hated or rejected because of our fat.

There is enough scientific evidence now to conclude that if we as fat people develop high blood pressure it is not because of our weight. It is because of what society does to intimidate, frighten and ostracise us. But, you may say, even if this is the reason, aren't we still going to die prematurely no matter what the *cause* of the high blood pressure? Dr Reubin Andres of the American National Institute of Ageing has reviewed the evidence from sixteen carefully controlled medical studies conducted in America and Europe. The result: 'It is concluded that the major studies of obesity and mortality fail to show that overall obesity leads to greater risk.'

In one study of middle-aged Swedish women, the death rate actually fell steadily with increasing fatness, even at the upper extremes of obesity.[6]

The world's largest ever epidemiological study was carried out on the population of Norway, monitoring 1.8 million participants over ten years.[7] The highest death rate occurred in underweight women, with those of 7st. 2lb and under at 5'3" being found twice as likely to die as women who were over 4st. heavier. The lowest mortality rate of all was amongst those who were approximately 30 per cent overweight. But even the women considered 'morbidly obese' had lower death rates than the underweight group. Some adversaries of this evidence tried to explain away the underweight deaths as being caused by smoking; in every controlled study the hazards of underweight were found to be equal in smokers and non-smokers.[8]

Dr Ernsberger[9] predicted life expectancy on the evidence of the Norwegian study. Out of four different weight groups of women aged thirty-five, our cultural and media 'heroine' — 5'7" and weighing 7st. 12lb — has the shortest life expectancy, with only 730 women in a thousand living until the age of 65. The woman weighing what she 'should' — 8st. 10lb — the 'insurance ideal' gives us a surprising result in terms of our conditioned beliefs; out of one thousand of these women, only 824 will live to age 65. The most surprising figure of all is that in the fat women group — those who weigh sixteen stones (225 lb) at 5'7" — 844 of the thousand will reach 65, the highest life expectancy of the group. And the 'morbidly obese' group, weighing more than twenty stones have a greater life expectancy than the thinnest, with 757 surviving till 65.

I spoke to Dr Celia Oakley, a consultant cardiologist at the Hammersmith Hospital in London. I asked her to give me the facts on the link between heart disease and overweight; her concise reply was that if you are overweight but do not have high blood pressure, high blood fats or diabetes, there is no associated risk. The qualifications to that are that to be morbidly obese (you know, she said, when you have to weigh people on the potato scales, when they really cannot even get out of bed) does carry risk of life and health. The other factor which incurs risk is to be substantially overweight when you already have diagnosed high blood pressure, diabetes or high blood fat. She also said that weight loss, even in the very obese, should be at the rate of about half a pound per week.

LIFE-STYLE AND HEALTH

It suggests to me, in the light of the cross-cultural evidence, that with our Western high fat diet it is a more than plausible possibility that *if* fat people are more prone to CHD it may well be that they have become fat, or fatter than they are meant to be, *not* by overeating, but by eating too much food rich in fat. It is quite difficult not to eat a high fat diet even if you are vegetarian. Apart from the obvious sources like fatty meat, milk and cheese, butter and eggs, there are sauces and dressings, spreads, cake, pastry, biscuits, crisps and some nuts. Many people are under the illusion that saturated fat means animal fat; unfortunately it also means hydrogenated vegetable fat and turns up in the most unlikely foods. Anything which says it contains vegetable fat is likely to contain the saturated variety. Brazil nuts and some shellfish are a particularly rich source of this unwanted type of fat.

Ah, but . . . often runs the argument against this . . . my grandfather lived until he was 93 and he had a farm and ate nothing but meat, milk, eggs, cheese and butter. This oft-repeated dismissal, usually trotted out by people who resent being told that research has discovered that their life-style and eating patterns may be harming their health, has truth in it.

The main points in this argument are the two important differences in late twentieth-century life-style compared with that of our grandparents which affect both our blood fats and our general fitness. The first is the dramatic decrease in physical exercise. We have become a sedentary nation. We rely on cars, to the point where our cities are clogged with permanent traffic jams and our atmosphere is dangerously polluted. We don't walk. We use lifts and elevators instead of stairs, hoovers instead of brooms, spray polish instead of beeswax and elbow grease. Technology works overtime to develop more and more products that will save us energy. We don't even beat up a cake with a wooden spoon now, we sling the ingredients into a food processor. There is even a machine for kneading bread. We 'go for a walk' as a kind of treat, at Christmas or on a sunny spring day. It is an event; we prepare for it and set off, consciously 'doing' something.

Even in a generation the difference shows. I and the other children where I lived had a mile to walk every day to school. I had to walk two miles to the nearest village for my mother nearly every day after school. My children and their friends protest at such an idea but it is not their fault, they are being brought up in a generation where, without even thinking about it, children are ferried about in cars by their parents.

It is not as black and white as that, of course. We have to consider our children's safety to a far greater extent nowadays and we don't have the rural buses that we used to. Nevertheless, our society is geared to taking our feet from under us and sitting us firmly down.

The other major influence on our cardiac health is twentieth-century stress. We live under the stress of work, of driving ourselves to achieve, of feeling failures if we do not, of taking on more than the human organism can cope with, of trying to combine careers with family life — and this applies to high-achieving men as well as women though naturally the pressure on women is far greater. There is the stress of competitiveness now being thrust upon our children, who do not rebel against the establishment any more because they are too busy trying to do well so that they can gain qualifications and avoid unemployment. And there is the stress of unemployment itself, poor housing; yes, I know there has always been poor housing but set in the context of our present day affluence the have-nots are far more disadvantaged than they used to be, because the very affluence of this society with its pride in its economy implies a deliberate and immoral lack of care for those who live in appalling conditions. And there is the environment which gets sicker and more damaged, bringing both the stress of environmental illness and the worry of wanting to do something to improve it without having the support of the whole world in doing so. Not to mention the ever-present fears about nuclear matters, whether it is waste, leaks or the weapons themselves.

Obesity has been wrongly indicted as a major health problem . . . This evil view of obesity has come from four places: the insurance industry, the medical moralisers (usually themselves thin), the drug industry, and the docile, unquestioning nutritionists who are too often dupes of the faddists and the hucksters.

Mann, G.V., 'Obesity the nutritional spook', 1971, in Ernsberger and Haskew, *Rethinking Obesity*, New York, 1987

Lack of exercise and stress both increase our blood fat levels whether or not we are fat. The fat person constantly lives under two major additional causes of stress — stigma and dieting.

It is important to bear in mind that the people who produce reports warning us of the dangers of being fat are nearly always doctors. According to Paul Ernsberger, a biomedical researcher on obesity, 'a particularly virulent form of fat bigotry seems to be endemic amongst physicians.'[10] And Natalie Allon, a sociologist who has spent much of her working life researching attitudes to fat people says that some medical doctors' condemnations of overweight in the name of disease really mask their moral and aesthetic biases. When we get into the area of the discrimination fat people suffer in society, we find that much of the damage to self-esteem and self-worth has been caused by doctors, many of whom treat fat people with contempt, disgust and punishment by refusing treatment until the patient has lost weight.[11]

Great Britain has the highest incidence of heart disease in the world, with Scotland the highest in Britain. The British Heart Foundation (BHF) spends a great deal of money on advertising and literature to inform people about heart disease and ways to improve their life-style in order to have a healthy heart. They produced an attractive looking series of informative pamphlets called the Heart Research Series, each one of which discusses in detailed, lay language different aspects of the heart and its diseases and mal-functions. 'Reducing the risk of a heart attack' is the one most health-conscious individuals picked out. It deals with all the risks to the heart. The small section on 'Obesity' is terse and to the point: 'There is little doubt that people who become substantially overweight before middle age and who then stay overweight are more likely to die prematurely'. Its advice, baldly put, is to lose weight.

The booklet also mentions the contraceptive pill as a heart attack risk, which is increased if you are over thirty-five, smoke or have a family history of heart disease. Occasionally there are scares about the pill reported in the papers, but I know several women over thirty-five who have been on the pill for a long time and who smoke. They seem to be treated with consideration by their doctors and family planning clinics, and if they wish to remain on the pill, great care and time is taken to find a lower dosage pill, a safer alternative, even though it still carries a risk. When I once said to a doctor at an obesity clinic that I had tried but failed to lose weight he said: 'I don't believe you have tried. You've just got to get on and do it. It's no different from taking medicine for the rest of your life — now just go away and do it.' This does not account for the 98 per cent failure in maintaining weight loss.

The BHF did not discuss at any length the issues of smoking, diet and blood pressure in its general pamphlets. Each was given a pamphlet to itself. But obesity had no pamphlet. This would seem to suggest that fatness is of lesser importance in the prevention of a heart attack than the other factors. If this is the case, why are fat people hounded and hassled so much by doctors? Or is it that what is seen as a self-inflicted condition is not considered worth a whole pamphlet?

The booklet on Familial Hyperlipidaemia (FH) (inherited high level of blood fats) advised that 'All FH patients should be on a low cholesterol, low saturated fat diet from early childhood. They should never smoke nor take contraceptive pills without medical advice'. It went on to discuss treatment for this condition with drugs or operations. There was no mention that these very high-risk people should avoid getting fat. A spokesman for the British Heart Foundation did not provide a conclusive answer to this omission.

In a study of adults in the Minneapolis–St. Paul area over the past few years, it was determined that heart disease has been on the decline, as has blood cholesterol, high blood pressure and smoking in the test subjects. However, the same subjects, on the average, got *fatter* over the test period.

From paper presented at the annual Conference on Heart Disease
Epidemiology, 1990, USA

Another BHF booklet, called *Diet and Your Heart*, was well set out and useful, defining saturated fats, fibre, polyunsaturated fats and unrefined carbohydrates. Its guidelines were good and I would certainly recommend the dietary advice. But when addressing the fat sinner the language and style changed from the factual, easy and informative manner of the rest of the pamphlets to a rebuking, nannyish and personal one which clearly, and almost certainly unconsciously, shows the prejudice the writer felt towards fat people. Why else would he need to say that 'several small meals are better than one big gorge'? Would not 'than one big one' convey exactly the same information? And is there really any call for this snippet of personal advice in a booklet about diet and the heart: 'The scales are only one criterion: your comfort is another. You want to be able to run upstairs and do whatever is consistent with your age and occupation.' This, surely, is astonishing. Even if we were to accept the premise that fat leads to heart disease, what makes this writer think that fat people *cannot* run upstairs and do whatever is consistent with our age and occupation, whatever that means? The only things that we cannot do that are 'consistent . . .' are those that society prevents by stigmatisation, discrimination and hatred. Or do we give this writer the benefit of the doubt and assume that while ostensibly writing about diet and the heart, he is tacitly admitting that we are prevented not by our size, but by society?

Further reading makes it impossible to confer such a benefit on this doctor, for his own prejudice seeps through in the next paragraph; *his* feelings about fat projected onto us, written by him but attributed to the fat reader of his wise words:[12]

> You want to be able to wear clothes that are something better than the trappings of grotesquerie; and you want to get rid of the rolls and bulges of fat of which you are uneasily or disgustedly aware.

Considering this is meant to be about health, the phrase 'trappings of grotesquerie' would take some beating in the most vitriolic condemnation of fat people. It is a wonderfully clear illustration, however, of the way the majority of physicians perceive us, and it should be borne in mind when reading or hearing about the health perils of being fat.

That is not to say that there is *no* health risk attached to being fat, but it must be put into perspective along with all the risks to our health we incur simply by living in the twentieth century.

Take smoking. If being fat is so aesthetically unappealing, what about

> brown stained fingers, hacking cough, dull grey complexion, grainy, coarse skin, vertical lines around the mouth, deeper frown and eye lines from squinting through cigarette smoke and yellow, stained teeth. And if you get close, clothes will smell of stale tobacco smoke, breath will smell like an ashtray and the voice may have a smoker's rasp to it.[13]

But smokers have not been perceived as socially unacceptable until very recently, and even now it is because of the recognized risks to other people's health and comfort. The glamorous image that smoking has carried for so many years is an enduring one, though; it will not be easy to stamp out. Despite government health warnings, smoking is not dying out. In fact, according to Neil Crawford, a psychotherapist at the Tavistock Centre, 'some people smoke *because* it is unacceptable . . . smoking is often a show of rebelliousness and individuality'.[14] I have never heard of anyone deliberately becoming fat in order to rebel against imposed thinness or to establish their individuality.

Company magazine interviewed three women smokers in their twenties. One, a public relations consultant, felt that smoking was part of her chosen image. She associates smokers with fun and lively sociable people:

> The brand you smoke is important. Benson and Hedges and Rothmans seem very male to me, I associate Marlboro with real macho smokers and Silk Cut is sophisticated and female . . . I never ask people who are still eating if I may smoke — they may say no . . . over half the cigarettes I smoke I don't enjoy. Sometimes they make me feel dizzy and sick. I understand what smoking is doing to me . . . but I completely blank out the health risks.

Other observations in the article were that smoking is a social bond and that even with health awareness, smoking seems to have a kind of Hollywood glamour about it; Lauren Bacall looks so sophisticated smoking. There is something special about having an engraved silver lighter, a fancy designer ashtray or even a cigarette holder.

The health risks are far more identifiable than with obesity and far more directly linked, from bronchitis through to emphysema, lung cancer and other cancers. But this is not deterring new women smokers; for the first time in smoking history, 16-29-year-old women smokers outnumber men in the same age group while the number of 20-24-year-old women smokers has stayed the same despite an overall national downward trend in the last ten years.

Nurses come into the 16-30 age group and see the results of cigarette smoking in their work. Yet there is a very high smoking rate in the nursing profession. I spoke to several nurses from different hospitals; all confirmed that a large proportion of their profession smoked. Why, when they knew the risks? Well, nursing is a high-stress job and smoking is a response to that. The alternative is that they find themselves eating through the combination of stress, the fast pace and the physical hard work. And nurses, like most women, are terrified of getting fat. In fact, apart from social reasons, nurses are not allowed to be fat, and there is a maximum weight requirement for student nurses in many hospitals. For example, St George's Hospital, London, will not accept a student who is more than 30 per cent above the standard height/weight ratio tables.

The fact that men appear to be giving up smoking in far greater numbers than women would suggest that women choose the smoker's health risk (and premature death) rather than the risk of getting fat. When a friend of mine joyfully announced to her friends that pregnancy had made smoking easy to give up as she had developed an aversion to it, she was met, not with their gladness at that news, but with a horrified 'But aren't you afraid you'll put on weight?' My mother, a smoker since the age of nineteen, was terrified of giving up on account of her fear of fatness. She developed cancer and emphysema in her fifties and gave it up simply because she was unable to breathe. Yes, she did put on weight; she went from a size 12 to a 14. Giving up was a terrible struggle; nicotine is as addictive as heroin and she did 'cold turkey'. Then she discovered her sense of smell and taste and started enjoying her food. But her heart was weakened by the emphysema and the cancer was advancing. She died at the age of 62, from a combination of diseases directly related to smoking. A friend's mother died of heart disease a few years before my mother. She too had been terrified of getting fat and would not consider giving up smoking. She was never a pound overweight, but she developed heart disease and died from it.

Kim Chernin[15] cites a telling example of our readiness to dispense with our health in order to lose weight. A friend of hers was taken to hospital suffering from abdominal pains so severe that she cried out; they were worse than the contractions of labour. After several days during which she was unable to eat, hospital staff brought scales into her room. She jumped onto them eagerly, impatiently awaiting the result and announced triumphantly that she had lost four and a half pounds. When she came home with the condition still undiagnosed, but with a question mark over abdominal cancer, the first thing she did was to check her five pound weight loss on her own scales. She told Kim Chernin that she would *like* to be able to say that she would willingly gain back the five pounds rather than go through 'that horrible pain again'. But she couldn't honestly say that was true. Later, when the horrors of her illness had been recounted at a dinner, two of her friends came up to her and said that there was a bright side to her illness: she had managed to lose five pounds. Kim Chernin says that none of these women was deranged; on the contrary, by the standards used to measure psychological adjustment they came out well.

Dr Jill Welbourne is a psychiatrist who has worked with (mostly) women with eating disorders for eighteen years in a Bristol hospital.[16] Most of her patients are anorexic; some are 'successful starvers' which means that they just do not eat; some of them are anorexic/bulimic. Some of them are also addicted to exercise which is another variation of the disorder. Jill Welbourne cites one patient, a married woman aged twenty-seven with three children who was of normal weight. She was eating a great deal of food, 3500–4000 calories a day, and doing nine aerobics classes and running twenty-six road miles for marathon training per week. Nothing wrong with that at first glance; running is a popular sport for women now and she would need to eat a great many calories in order not to lose too much weight and stamina. But the nine aerobics classes are a give-away. She was in fact addicted to exercise to the extent that she had a psychological disorder. This was revealed when she broke her pelvis. Her disproportionate distress at not being able to run revealed her problem to her GP.

Exercise and fasting, or depriving yourself of food — as fasting has positive moral and spiritual connotations — both release endorphins in the brain which cause the sort of 'high' experienced by drug abusers. That is why they are addictive. Like cream cakes — 'naughty, but nice'; though can you imagine anyone wagging a reproving finger at someone eating too little or taking a great deal of exercise? Concern, we've all heard it (directed towards others!): 'I'm worried about you; you're not eating enough' — compared with rebuke: 'You'll get fat eating that', or 'Your eyes are bigger than your stomach'.

Social and cultural hostility towards fatness shows this

clear line between care and concern on behalf of the thin child/adolescent/ woman and reproach, censure and disapproval for the fat child or woman. This affects the way we are treated; it is defined by our body size and our eating habits from the earliest age. A mother will show concern over her twelve year old who never seems to eat a proper meal, but a child who grows fat will soon be made aware, at school or in the street that 'thou shalt not get fat' is one of the first laws of social integration and acceptability.

A fat child may be taken, or a fat woman may take herself, to a clinic for eating disorders, or help may be sought from her GP; she may even attend one of the specialist obesity clinics. What she will observe, consciously or otherwise, is that those who are too thin, who do not eat enough, will receive medical care of a nurturing kind. This is not usually available to the fat sinner, who can only earn approval by proving she will lose weight.

This area is full of medical paradoxes. We who are fat are told we are in danger of everything from arthritis to heart disease to sudden premature death. If we are very overweight, the helpful pamphlets suggest that we need help urgently. To get the help is another thing entirely. The GP will give us a diet sheet; most fat women know more than most GPs about diets. My local clinic for weight problems and eating disorders has closed its doors to fat people — it is full to overflowing with anorexics. Yet only about 1 per cent of all anorexics in Britain die from the condition.[17] So if it is so life-threatening and unhealthy to be fat, why are we not being offered supportive medical help? What is the real truth about fat health and thin health?

Jill Welbourne, who has treated underweight women and overweight women, all with a variety of different emotional problems, is unequivocal. 'Being thin is what kills you,' she says. And she is prepared to put herself on the line for her controversial observations, based on many years of specialising, that the largest group of women with eating disorders are those who are not generally recognized as sick; i.e. not the obese nor the anorexic, but the women of average weight whose obsession with remaining 'normal' takes over their lives. These are the women who would naturally be a little heavier if they lived a normal life-style; but they do not. They are the successful dieters, the Weight Watchers addicts, the ones whose conversation invariably turns to weight control, the women who insist that they are fat when they are clearly not, who talk about their 'gross thighs' or stomachs or hips, thus drawing attention to perfectly average sized or shaped portions of their anatomy. These are the women whose remarks in the presence of food are as ritualised as the saying of grace and always predictable: 'Think of the calories in this'; 'Oh no, I never eat pudding, I have to watch my figure — if I don't nobody else will.'

These, too, are the women who, while not being bulimic, by definition have jumped on the bandwagon of bulimia. If they have eaten a larger meal than they would have liked, at a business lunch or a calorie-laden wedding reception, they will repair to the ladies cloakroom, stick their fingers down their throats and bring up the unwanted calories.

I watched a television documentary some years ago on the dangers of this new disease, bulimia nervosa. The commentary explained how dangerous it was; that self-induced vomiting caused physical problems, from swollen salivary glands in the neck to teeth stripped of their enamel, and that the very real danger was to the heart. Induced vomiting causes muscle spasms which can affect the heart muscle, and a complete imbalance of the blood electrolytes including a dangerous deficiency of potassium; both these things can lead to arrhythmia and cardiac arrest. Then a woman was interviewed. She was beautifully dressed and groomed and she told her story. Some years ago, she said, she had weighed sixteen stones (225lb) and had not been able to diet successfully. Then she heard of bulimia and now weighed nine stones (126lb), through practising regular vomiting. No, she would not dream of giving it up, in spite of knowing the risks, because life simply was not worth living at sixteen stones, while at nine all her dreams were coming true.

I talked to a friend of mine, one whom I knew to be obsessive about her (normal) weight and who had to attend a large number of professional lunches and dinners. Did she know of women who vomited up their meals to prevent weight gain, I asked her? Did *she* do it? Of course, she said, seeming rather surprised at my question. Doesn't everyone?

These normal weight women are sick because their raison d'etre is dependent on constant and perfect control. This leaves no room in their lives for normal thinking, normal unfettered living. They cannot let go, even for a day, of the restricting self-discipline that binds any real freedom of expression with a tight cord, because those who are abnormally bound in one area are not able to be truly free in others; they are unlikely to be able to throw off their chains in order to enjoy other sensual pleasures. And it has been recognized for a very long time that food and sex are inseparably intertwined; you cannot mortify your fleshly desires in one area and joyfully free them in another.

I read an article in *Weight Watchers.*[18] It had the most marvellous illustration depicting the fat woman as sinner that I have ever seen. There she stands on a pair of scales, sprouting two horns and the classic devil's tail. There are two diaphanous (thin!) angels hovering by her head, each holding a large tape measure which both bear such legends as 'diabetes, coronary artery disease, hyperlipidaemia' and other familiar tales. I cannot make out whether the angels are proffering these as warnings or as a means of salvation; I suppose it comes to the same in the end — repent, using the tape measure as your bible, and you shall be saved (from high blood pressure etc.). They appear to be whispering in her ear; the dietary secrets of eternal life, perhaps?

Having been utterly enchanted by this pictorial, and therefore clearly stated illustration of us sinners as seen by the world, I found the article to be the usual litany of warnings about the health perils of being fat. But for the first time in an article of this sort, the writer admits that these diseases are not caused by overweight. They are aggravated by them. That is why, says the article, slightly disapprovingly, some doctors will not insist that an overweight person diets, even if they are quite severely overweight, unless they have a family history of these conditions. (Where are these doctors? They should be shared out amongst all the hundreds of fat women who have spoken so unhappily about the harsh and dismissive attitudes of their GPs. I thought I had the only good one.)

FAT
- There is no known cause for obesity
- There is no known cure
- Obese people do not on the average eat more than anyone else
- Ninety per cent of Americans who lose weight through dieting gain it back within two years
- There is little scientific evidence to prove that obesity causes high blood pressure or heart disease
- Slightly overweight people live longer than thin people
- Taking amphetamines, fasting, undergoing gastric stapling or constantly gaining and losing weight are dangerous to your health.

Poster in the Smithsonian Museum, Washington DC, displayed in an exhibition titled 'Clothes, Gender and Power', which included a section on diet products.

This is an admission of no small significance, especially in a slimming magazine. Of course it does go on to say that we should lose weight lest we develop these illnesses, without even paying lip-service to the fact that doctors themselves do not have the answer to the 98 per cent weight gain after dieting. You can at any time choose to change your life-style, the writer says blithely.

The article starts to talk some real sense when it mentions the American magazine *Radiance* which 'defies most medical wisdom linking obesity and illness'. *Radiance* questions why no one highlights the fact that thin people have an increased cancer risk and are more likely to get emphysema and TB and suffer from ulcers, anaemia, brittle bones and give birth to underdeveloped babies. The article also quotes *Radiance* as insisting that 'the fat person who eats well and gets lots of exercise may be healthier than the thin person who doesn't'. But after this glimpse of enlightening insight and wisdom, the moralising returns:

> Despite the efforts of this movement to try and inject a positive image of fat people, the fact is that over-eating is a symptom of an unbalanced lifestyle — and one must expect effects on one's health which will get worse as one gets older.

Unbalanced life-style. I am reminded of 'the trappings of grotesquerie'. Wherever we look we encounter the assumptions which are made about fat people — their eating habits, their slovenliness, their inability to look good or perform well in any area of life — and so the stereotype is constantly reinforced. While researching this book, I have delved deep into medical, sociological and psychological studies, surveys and books on the effects of being large, fat, overweight, big, heavy, or whatever description you prefer. It would be impossible to summarise the findings in a single chapter on health, but there are facts that all fat people should know. To list them may seem inadequate, but they will give you clear information to use — for yourself, because you have the right to know the truths; for combating medical prejudice or refusal of treatment; and for dealing with the accusations, taunts and so-called helpful advice from the world in general. All these facts are substantiated by research, most of it going back over a period of many years. I am indebted to Dr Jill Welbourne of the Bristol Royal Infirmary, Dr Celia Oakley of Hammersmith Hospital, London, Dr Paul Ernsberger of Cornell University, New York, Drs Wayne and Susan Wooley of University of Cincinnati, and Paul Haskew, Ed.D, Psychologist, University of Connecticut — all of whom contributed to disentangling fact from myth.

The truth

Moderate obesity, that is about two stones (30lb) over the height/ weight chart limit, is healthier than thinness.

Obesity *per se* is not a major risk factor in coronary heart disease or premature death, though extreme obesity may pose a threat if there is *existing* heart disease or hyperlipidaemia (high blood fat).

No study has reported a direct relationship between overweight and death from all causes, or from coronary heart disease.

The incidence of atherosclerosis in coronary and other vessels is entirely unrelated to body fatness, as autopsies have demonstrated.

The prognosis for survival from coronary heart disease may be more favourable in fat than in lean people.

High blood pressure and coronary heart disease occurs in thin and fat people, and many other factors have to be taken into account: heredity, smoking, diet and life-style.

A substantial number of studies have shown that there is a lower mortality rate in fat people with high blood pressure than in thin or average-weight persons.

Substantial overweight may lead to late-onset diabetes, though it would appear that the obesity-linked type of diabetes is less complicated and carries less risk than the genetically-predisposed type.

Fat people experience lower incidences of most cancers than thin or normal-weight people; this also applies to lung diseases, bone diseases and certain heart conditions.

Fat women have a much lower incidence of fractures and osteoporosis; hip fracture is the greatest cause of disability in American women and a major cause of death.

Fat people have a more efficient immune system and therefore they are less prone to infectious diseases.

Their recovery rate is better so overall fatalities from infectious diseases are lower.

They have a lower suicide rate.

The incidence of wound infection may be greater after surgery.

Arthritis may be exacerbated by weight, though not necessarily caused by it.

Fat women are less likely to suffer from pregnancy eclampsia, premature birth, vaginal laceration during delivery, early menopause and hot flushes (fat cells store oestrogen, the hormone that is depleted at menopause).

Endometrial cancer is more prevalent in fat women, probably because of the greater stores of oestrogen; however it is one of the most easily detectable and curable cancers.

In some circumstances, treatment of obesity carries greater risk than the condition itself.

And finally — this is not to be taken lightly: DIETING SERIOUSLY DAMAGES YOUR HEALTH (see Chapter 8 for more detail).

The myths corrected

All available evidence suggests that there is nothing abnormal about the way fat people eat. Some are big eaters, some are not and the same is true of thin people. No one has been able to demonstrate that they eat too much, or eat the wrong foods — the 'stuffing themselves with cream cakes' myth.

Fat people do not take more time off work through illness than average-weight people.

Diets do not work.

Fitness and fatness are perfectly compatible.

Fat people are not of lower intelligence.

They do not sweat or smell more than average-weight people.

They do not necessarily have high blood pressure (in the United States tight cuffs were found to register a higher pressure; when bigger, more comfortable cuffs were used on large people, blood pressure was lower).

Pregnancy is not risky and fertility is not impaired (except in the excessively fat where hormonal changes may affect ovulation and menstruation; however, this happens more frequently in thin than in fat people).

Fat women can breastfeed successfully (I fed my three children for periods of one to three years).

Varicose veins are not more common, nor are fallen arches.

And, in surgery, where doctors and dietitians alike seem to take a perverse pleasure in terrifying fat people:

Fat embolism is very rare.

It is not more difficult to sew up fat tissue after an operation, it just takes longer and gives the surgeon more to do.

And, perhaps the most common threat made — it is not dangerous to give a fat person an anaesthetic. To be told to lose several stones before a surgeon will operate is blackmail. If you are thinner, it is easier for the doctor.

Every single diet results in a binge. It doesn't matter what you're on. Everyone who is involved with them knows they don't work.

Jane R. Hirschmann, co-author of *Overcoming Overeating* quoted in *The New York Times*, 5 January, 1990

Dr Jill Welbourne, who used to be an anaesthetist at St Mary's Hospital, London, told me:

> Of course doctors don't like giving anaesthetics to fat patients — it means they have to work harder! Yes, it is more difficult than with a person of normal weight, but there are all sorts of other variables. It's more difficult with smokers and drinkers too. The anaesthetic stays in the tissues for longer in fat people, so the anaesthetist has to watch the controls more carefully.
>
> When a fat person comes in for an anaesthetic, it's like reading a Dickens novel when you've been reading a string of Mills and Boon! You have to concentrate much harder!

8
To diet or not to diet?

Cardiac problems, gallstones, weakness, fatigue, gout, arthritis, disordered heartrate, oedema, aching muscles, abdominal pain, raised cholesterol, changed liver function, pancreatic complications, decreased libido — and the ultimate health disorder — death. A list of horrors with which the overweight will be all too familiar — after all, we've been threatened with them all our lives. This is our fate, we are told, if we do not mend our gluttonous ways and *diet*.

In fact the above conditions are just some of the risks of *dieting*, documented by Professor Janet Polivy of the University of Toronto who has been researching the effects of dieting since the early 1970s.[1] She is not alone. At the University of Cincinnati College of Medicine Eating Disorders Clinic, Dr Wayne and Dr Susan Wooley have recorded the same findings, and researchers Dr Paul Ernsberger and Dr Paul Haskew have collated hundreds of studies going back several decades. The conclusions support the evidence: dieting is not only hazardous, it can kill you. 'Yo-yo dieting' has been cited as dangerous. Right back in the 1960s in the United States, a physicians' desk-top guide, the *Merck Manual* stated: 'In patients who cannot maintain weight loss, obesity may be preferable to frequent wide fluctuations in weight, since atherosclerosis seems to be associated with such oscillations.'[2] Pioneers in the field of health, weight and dieting, such as Albert Stunkard and Ancel Keys, were demonstrating as far back as 1950 that dieting was damaging to the heart and other organs. Deaths from rigorous starvation diets were reported including that of a 17-year-old girl in a British hospital who suffered several cardiac arrests when she began the refeeding process, that is beginning to eat 'normally' again.[3] *The Lancet* reported in 1969 that: 'It seems that prolonged total starvation produces gross destruction of cardiac myofibrils and we suggest that this regimen should no longer be recommended as a safe means of weight reduction.'[4]

I could fill an entire book with the findings of the researchers who discovered decades ago what a hazardous business dieting was. But no one listened to them. While Britain and the United States continued to respond to the tyranny of the fat-hating medical profession, to the power of the diet industry and to the all-prevalent disease of socially induced dietmania, there was little chance of these lone voices being heard except by their own kind. And there were no signs that anything would halt the growing tide of diets, diet books and products, slimming clubs and constant, eroding pressure from all sides. In the United States, the National Association to Advance Fat Acceptance (NAAFA), the civil rights pressure group, grew in strength, but still remained a minority in a vast country. In Britain the successful National Fat Women's Conference of 1989 was never repeated, even though hundreds of women had been turned away, so great was the response. The London Fat Women's Group who had organised it so brilliantly seemed to fade away. Being fat, we are told, *is* a sin; and even those bookshops which proclaimed that they were feminist or politically sound displayed shelves laden with diet books.

COMES THE REVOLUTION?

In the early part of 1992 there was a shift in public consciousness. Newspapers carried reports of anti-diet demonstrations throughout the United States which were likened to the bra-burning protests of the early women's movement. In these latest demonstrations, women burned diet books and smashed bathroom scales. They carried banners which proclaimed: 'Scales are for fish, not for women.' Industries and health organizations suspended weight-loss programmes; the Houston oil giant, Cocono, replaced diet seminars for employers with 'Pleasure Principle Wellness',[5] a programme encouraging both men and women to respect their bodies, to work at self-acceptance, to eat in response to stomach hunger and to stay away from scales, fitness tests and highly structured exercise plans.

There were several major catalysts involved in this revolt. David Garner of Michigan State University and Susan Wooley from University of Cincinnati produced a 40-page report on 'the failure of behavioural and dietary treatments for obesity'. This report questioned why other studies which had repeatedly demonstrated the failure of diets were ignored, and the authors challenged the entire health-care profession's insistence that obesity carried significant risks which warranted weight reduction. They also pointed out that 'the commercial weight loss industry (is) now a major economic force in North America'. The data suggesting that obesity is a health risk, is, they said 'weak and conflicting'. The report, which is highly detailed, carries a clear message: there is no scientific justification for the continued use of dieting. It does not work. Weight lost will be regained.

In addition to demonstrating the complete uselessness of dieting, David Garner and Susan Wooley took a close look at some studies which suggested that weight loss actually increased the risk of premature death. Each one of these showed that those who dieted died earlier than those whose weight remained stable — *even if that weight was high*. Yo-yo dieting — now called weight recycling — was examined and found to be extremely hazardous; in one study quoted, those participants who had dieted and regained were *twice* as likely to die from cardiovascular disease than those who maintained a stable weight over 25 years.[6] The authors agreed with physiologist Ancel Keys that this was due to the high levels of blood cholesterol associated with weight regain.

In 1984, when Dr Susan and Dr Wayne Wooley asked the question: 'Should obesity be treated at all?' it was considered too shocking to be taken seriously and was largely ignored by the health community. But in March 1992 the American government tackled the issue at a National Institute of Health Conference on *Methods for Voluntary Weight Loss and Control*. Its conclusions, after hearing evidence, were: that weight-loss strategies have caused harm; weight lost is nearly always regained; weight recycling could be harmful; the media present unrealistic role models which people try to emulate; many Americans who are not overweight are dieting and most major studies suggest increased mortality is associated with weight loss.

It's taken a long time. In the 1960s, William Fabrey, co-founder of NAAFA, said:

There are important questions which should be investigated before any organisation attempts to prescribe diet as a means of increasing one's life span. Wouldn't it be ironic if the American preoccupation with dieting *decreases* the life span of more people than it increases! I feel this may be a distinct possibility.[7]

Prophetic words which went unheeded for 30 years, along with the work done by the researchers who *knew* they had got it right. But with the endorsement of the American government following Garner and Wooley's report, *some* doctors and *some* minds are opening at last.

THE ANTI-DIET MOVEMENT

If this is a revolution, America and Canada were not only at its vanguard, they were ahead of it. NAAFA, founded in 1969, has made its voice heard right across the United States. More than an anti-diet movement, it crusades actively and politically on behalf of fat Americans, and has a number of respected medical professionals on its board. NAAFA has clout — it is out to change the world (at least the American world) and it is doing more than just making waves.

Since 1988, Health and Welfare Canada have had a policy advocating the promotion of good eating, the importance of environment and life-style and the acceptance of a broad range of weights. Health professionals were issued a clear directive: 'If you cannot help, at least do no harm', an aphorism I would like to see in every doctor's surgery, office or consulting room to remind them what their vocation is really about — a consideration which tends to go by the board when a large-size patient walks into their domain. Canada also has a nationwide programme called 'Vitality', which aims to promote health by encouraging people to feel good about themselves and their bodies, eat well and be active, and accept that health does not necessarily mean slimness. There are also courses designed to break the diet habit and mentality. They run for 10 to 12 weeks and focus on self-esteem, dealing with the cultural pressure to be thin, and 'deprogramming' people from the ever-present obsession with food and weight.

Groups like these are emerging in Britain with varying degrees of reticence, by which I mean they are far from household names like Weight Watchers — with one exception. In the early part of 1992, management consultant Mary Evans Young founded 'Dietbreakers'. Mary is a warm, comfortable woman, not fat, but certainly overweight by perceived standards of the ideal body. She is done with dieting once and for all and she is a dynamic campaigner. Within weeks of its inception, the name Dietbreakers was everywhere. Women, she said, brooking no argument, *must* free themselves from the tyranny of dieting and put a stop to the growing power of the slimming industry in all its guises. The first 'National No Diet Day' was organised by Mary and took place on 5th May 1992 in London's Hyde Park where a group of women celebrated with a picnic. By 5th May 1993, it had become International No Diet Day with a press conference at the House of Commons, guest speakers and an Early Day Motion tabled by Labour MP Alice Mahon. This called for an end to the pressure to diet and the introduction of legislation curtailing the diet industry. Mary's energy and commitment are boundless and No Diet Day 1993 was truly international, being celebrated across America and Canada as well. Those participating or supporting wore pale blue ribbons, and good food was enjoyed and eaten without guilt or inhibition. This date has been set for all future International No Diet Days. Knowing Mary as I do, I confidently predict that Dietbreakers will nip sharply at the heels of the slimming clubs, causing them to look behind themselves with some well justified misgivings.

Dietbreakers produces a newsletter for its members and Mary Evans Young has been working with Linda Omichinski, a Canadian nutritionist who for some time has run a successful anti-diet course in Canada, called HUGS. The title of Linda's book — *You Count, Calories Don't* — encapsulates the HUGS philosophy of building self-worth and breaking the dieting stranglehold. HUGS, incidentally, is not an acronym. Linda says it is simply because she wants women to feel that hugs are what they deserve, whether physical, metaphorical or symbolic — treats, in other words, demonstrations of love and approval. We can give them to ourselves in the form of self-acceptance and affirmation of our own worth, and we can be taught to believe we are worthy of receiving the same kind of treatment from others. It's the perhaps trite principle of loving yourself, but in the case of Linda's HUGS programme it has restored a sense of worth and validity to many women. Now Mary is co-ordinating HUGS in the UK.

Because I know Mary and Linda, I can recommend them and their work in the anti-diet movement to anyone who is caught on the treadmill of self-disgust, on-off dieting and low self-worth. More than that, I would recommend them to anyone who does *not* suffer self-loathing but who has reached self-acceptance and confidence *only* through meticulous, unremitting control of her weight. As long as you believe that your worth, your success, your ability to make relationships work or wear nice clothes depends on being *slim*, you are a victim, as much in need of anti-diet help as those whose size makes them feel they only dare face the world if they are showing awareness of their sin by dieting.

There are friends of mine (mentioning no names but they will recognize themselves), who fulsomely praised the first edition of this book, who said how much it was doing for large women, who passionately insisted that there was a *need* for such a book. Most of these friends are committed *feminists* and they are very slim. Not naturally so, but by a combination of dietary vigilance and the same kind of horror of getting fat that makes (most) sexually active people condom-conscious because of the fear of AIDS. You think I'm exaggerating, perhaps. Believe me, it's true. I have ceased to be amazed at the number of campaigning, crusading, politically conscious feminists who have a copy of *The Hip and Thigh Diet* on their bookshelves. 'I think what you are doing is wonderful' they say to me (subtext: '*As long as I don't get fat like you*'). If I suggest they join Dietbreakers they either look nervous or guilty, or they take themselves off to the next Weight Watchers meeting — 'because I would just like to lose half a stone'.

I'm not being as censorious as I sound. Of course I can understand why no one in this society would want to get fat — the pain and punishment of doing so are too great. What does make me angry is the women who persist in keeping themselves a size 10 or 12 — maybe 14 if they are tall. 'Oh no,' they say to me, 'I wouldn't mind putting on a bit of weight — it's just that I don't want to have to go out and buy a whole new wardrobe.' This response is so predictable that I can say, after their declaration that they wouldn't mind putting on the weight, 'Yes, I know. But you don't want to have to go out and buy a whole new lot of clothes.' They look quite surprised at my apparent perspicacity. Funny how women who *lose* weight are always *delighted* when they have to buy a new lot of (smaller) clothes! Very consistent, this pattern. How often do you hear women say that they must lose a few pounds because their skirts are tight? How often do you hear them say they must *gain* a few pounds because their skirts have become too loose? And I'm talking about 'normal' weight women.

BEWARE OF THE BANDWAGON

The rise of anorexia, the public forum of bulimia (it seems that every female celebrity is now coming out in women's magazines and saying 'I was Bulimic' in 'True Confessions' style), and the awareness of the real dangers of dieting have all combined to convince a large slice of the medical profession that a 'mild' degree of overweight is preferable to 'weight recycling'. Newspapers, radio and television in Britain have featured doctors who have said that their real concern is the number of women who do not really need to lose weight but who are diet-obsessed. And Mary Evans Young has found that the majority of dieting women only want to lose a maximum of ten pounds. While the anti-diet movement is long overdue, and the best thing since the women's movement and the Equal Opportunities Commission, it has some disadvantages for large-size women. While in no way intending to diminish the importance of the movement, I just feel that we should exercise a degree of caution in certain areas.

Many anti-diet books and courses are still promoting and offering weight loss. 'Lose weight without dieting' is the catchphrase to beware of, and since the awareness of the dangers of dieting you will see this slogan replacing many of those coverlines on women's magazines that promise wonderful, new, exciting diets. The courses run by Mary Evans Young and Linda Omichinski do not offer you weight loss, but some of these new-wave organizations will be doing just that. We need to remember that where there is a new trend of any sort there will be entrepreneurs who will profit from it. I have had details of no-diet programmes which claim to re-educate you so that you are 'in control of your eating', and by so doing you will find the weight dropping off. One of these lasts for four days and costs in the region of £200. Women, desperate to lose weight and knowing in their hearts that they have failed to do so by dieting, are terribly susceptible to this new propaganda. If they only stopped to give it some thought they would realize that there *is* no magic formula which in only four days will enable them to lose weight in a different, new way. What they will lose is a lot of money.

What troubles me greatly is that the anti-diet movement provides another bandwagon and one in which integrity is compromised. Apart from exceptions, like Mary and Linda, there are still no signs that fat acceptance is becoming a reality. There is a great deal of tokenism going on. Let me give an example. In January 1992, before the UK movement existed, I took part in a radio discussion with journalist Vanessa Feltz, then writing for *Slimmer* Magazine. I said that women were driven blindly to dieting. Vanessa Feltz replied emphatically:

> 'It's because we're *not* blind that we're driven to dieting. Slimness is attractive. Slimness is sexy. Fat actively interferes with a fulfilling sex life — I don't know if you know this — luckily I haven't had to experience it.'
> 'Rubbish' I said.
> 'It is actually *not rubbish*' protested V. Feltz. 'Fat ladies are sometimes reduced to sticking pillows under their behinds in order that the right bit will rub against the right bits effectively. Also, if you feel fat and you know that when you take your bra or girdle off all your vital statistics will plummet dramatically towards your feet, you possibly don't feel sexy or attractive and find it difficult to recline and enjoy the attentions of your lover. This is *definitely* the case and surveys all over the country will prove this.'

I went on to say that large women do have a fulfilling sex life, that men are responsive to flesh and don't like sharp bones sticking in them and that I had had women confiding in me that they were embarrassed about their naked *thin* bodies, their tiny flat breasts, their bones sticking out. After a bit more discussion with a young actress also taking part, Feltz returned to her theme: 'Sex *does* very largely depend on physical attraction, i.e. what the other person looks like. After all, it's the first thing you notice about someone . . . and if they're fat and their bits are hanging out it's unlikely that you're going to want to go over and embrace them. That is fact.'

The June 1993 issue of *She* magazine carried two main cover lines: 'Stop dieting and lose weight' and 'Very big can be very, very sexy.' This second article was titled 'I'm big and I'm sexy', with the subtitle 'Men like large women, says Vanessa Feltz'. 'I could do with losing a couple of stone' she begins, and carries on by describing herself — 'billowing mush . . . stretch marked flaps of belly, a second chin (which) spreads out under the first like a Hovercraft cushion . . .' and so on. Then: 'That said, can I possibly think I'm sexy? Are you kidding? I know I am! A darned sight sexier now than when I fluttered on to the scales at eight stone four. Don't be so fattist.' She went on to say what I had said on the radio programme, that men *like* flesh. And — 'Of course, sex appeal hasn't got a lot to do with what you look like anyway.' Yes, it *was* the same Vanessa Feltz! Not a reformed Vanessa Feltz who had put on a couple of stones — I remember thinking on the day of the radio discussion that attractive though she was, her size made her an odd advertisement for *Slimmer* magazine. She and *She* were just climbing onto the current, anti-diet bandwagon.

The other article in that issue illustrates everything that makes me wary about the anti-diet movement. Entitled 'Why I don't diet any more', it shows a photograph of a slim woman, Sarah Clarke, who 'has freed both mind and body'. She tells a story of weight obsession — 'even a one pound difference in my weight drastically affected my mood' — and of repeated diets of all kinds. Now she has stopped dieting and is happy with herself and her weight.

Sounds fine, put like that. But Sarah Clarke, at 5'3" weighed 10½ stones (147lb) at her *heaviest*. We are not talking overweight here, or fat, or even plump. This article carries the signs of obsession: 'I can remember baking cakes every weekend, almost as an act of self-torture, and feeling pious when I mustered the willpower to resist a crumb. I can remember the back of my neck burning when I went up to the counter in the canteen at work for a stodgy pudding, convinced that people would be eyeing my figure from behind and thinking what a pig I was.' This woman now weighs eight stone five. She spends several hours a week exercising and I would challenge her assertion that she is freed in body and mind, because she is still focused on weight: 'I can maintain my weight and lose a few pounds if I want to.' Isn't this a contradiction in terms? She still feels self-conscious about some parts of her body and 'feel more comfortable covering them up even in the hottest weather but on the whole I view my body as a friend rather than a foe'. Another contradiction — if her body is a friend, why does she feel the need to cover it in hot weather at only eight stone five (119lb)?

This kind of anti-diet message is the one that is given such approval by the health-care professionals. These are the women who have an anorexic potential but who now feel that they have stopped dieting and halted the possible slide into an eating disorder. They are the natural size 12s who have agreed to stop forcing their bodies to be size 10s, and the tall, big-boned size 14s who have accepted that aiming at size 12 is not realistic.

This aspect of the anti-diet message puts women who are more than a couple of stones overweight by the charts into an impossible situation. In an article about compulsive eating, which gives acknowledgement and approval to NAAFA and Dietbreakers, the author says that: '. . . the idea is that when you forget about diets, you get to your "ideal" weight naturally. Success is when people say they haven't thought about food for a month, and they don't care that they're two pounds overweight'.[8] The complex nature of fatness itself means that very few large people will be able to lose weight in this over-simplistic way. For one thing, there is a growing body of evidence which points to obesity being genetic. This means that if someone who weighed more than average was *left alone* right from childhood and not forced to diet, she would probably stabilise at a much higher weight than is considered acceptable in our culture. However, she would be healthy. This rarely happens, though, because dieting is an ingrained part of Western social behaviour and children as young as five are now becoming weight conscious. Most 'normal' weight women diet at some point; it is highly improbable that someone whose weight was higher than average would have reached adulthood without having dieted several times.

There are many reasons for being overweight or fat or large, but the gluttony and slothfulness attributed to fat people is rarely the cause. Apart from the genetic factor, it is now indisputable that dieting makes you fat. Those with a predisposition to gain weight will have dieted many times, often losing and then regaining vast amounts, throwing their metabolism into chaos. The combined stress of this and the social persecution that we live under brings emotional and psychological factors into many large people's eating patterns. Fear of food — of what we believe it has done to us, and what we believe it will go on doing to us if we don't somehow learn to 'control' it — is a powerful force.

Fat people can be divided into two groups — those who have accepted that they will not lose weight and who have been able to make peace with food, and those who find the stigma and threats almost unendurable and keep trying, somehow, to 'do something about it'. Neither group is allowed to live in peace; even if you maintain a stable weight you will be persecuted, though the very fact of weight remaining stable is evidence that the individual cannot be indulging in any kind of gluttony! In this society, though, it is not enough to demonstrate, by the fact of not *gaining* weight, that you are not 'overeating'. You are required to deprive yourself so that you practise a sort of auto-cannibalism until the 'excess' weight goes.

What are we to do now that we are faced with a frightening array of medical paradoxes? The evidence is unambiguous — dieting is a threat to health and life. Yet we are not permitted by our medical profession to seek a healthy life-style *and* remain fat. We are told that we will suffer heart disease and early death, yet deaths previously attributed to excess weight have been more closely examined and many of these occur while dieting is taking place. We are denied operations and other forms of medical treatment. Doctors who predict fatal heart attacks are still largely of the opinion that Very Low Calorie Diets should be indicated in cases of 'severe obesity'. The very nature of VLCDs means that they cause rapid weight loss followed by regain when the diet is stopped — and it has been demonstrated that this period of regain is highly dangerous for the heart. Yet the British Heart Foundation recommends liquid diets of less than 600 calories a day for the 'severely obese'. The same applies to weight-loss surgery which cannot help but cause rapid weight loss. And why are we suitable candidates for *that* surgery, which necessitates an anaesthetic, when we are refused other kinds of operations?

We have a choice. To remain the weight and size we are and to keep in mind the research that suggests that there is no link between obesity and mortality but that there certainly is between dieting and mortality. Or to find a way of losing weight *very, very slowly and not to put it back*. Given the bleak figure that 95-98 per cent of weight lost is regained, the fat woman is now in a terrible dilemma. Sensitised by a lifetime of threats she must now face the knowledge that the one thing she kept up her sleeve as the means to salvation — dieting repeatedly — is no longer an option. But if she chooses to remain large, she will be harassed from all quarters. The fat woman now is truly caught between a rock and a hard place, and the stress caused by the double fear of remaining fat and of risking her life by dieting is likely to rise.

This is where the medical profession has failed us completely. Although not true in every case, the majority of fat women have a history of disordered eating which has been caused by dieting. What is not recognized is that this is often identical to that of the bulimic. The fat woman will talk of dieting and breaking her diet, the bulimic of bingeing and purging. It comes to the same thing. Like the anorexic and the bulimic, the fat woman loses touch with her body's messages. She cannot distinguish between emotional hunger and stomach hunger. She does not recognize satiety and her eating is often chaotic and out of control. Food seems dangerous. In the spectrum of eating disorders, while bulimics are 'failed' anorexics, the overweight dieters are the 'failed' bulimics. If any large woman reading this feels indignant at the suggestion that she may be suffering from an eating disorder, I would like to reassure her that experiments show that people who have only dieted *once* become obsessed with food. Dieting is starvation. You will hear people say with great sarcasm that fat people *must* overeat because, after all, no-one came out of Belsen fat. No, but many survivors of the concentration camps grew hugely fat afterwards — deprivation throws the body into a panic and it frantically lays down fat stores to prepare for the next famine. You cannot defeat your own physiology.

Yet none of this is acknowledged or recognized as a condition meriting therapy. The emotional, social and personal pressures which cause disordered eating and body weight need to be addressed in a therapeutic context so that, with help, the large woman can come to understand her deeper needs. Then she may or may not lose weight spontaneously. But on the whole this sort of therapy is only available to the anorexic and the bulimic. The harsh fact is that those who diet and binge then induce vomiting or abuse laxatives will be offered this kind of help, while those who diet and binge and *refrain* from abusing their body as the bulimic does, but puts on weight instead, will be censured, condemned, told to diet or offered risky, mutilating surgery.

I telephoned one London hospital with a renowned clinic for eating disorders. I asked about their methods and was told that patients were given extensive psychotherapy to help them to get to the root of their eating or weight problem. 'Fat people too?' I asked. No, was the reply, they are seen in the obesity clinic. Yes, it was true that they too needed psychotherapy and understanding but there just were not the resources. 'They are helped, though,' I was told. 'We do jaw wiring here and we're using a new method of stomach stapling.'

Committing the sin of getting fat excludes women from the kind of therapeutic care available to their anorexic and bulimic counterparts. I have a letter from a woman who found a way round this. After years of failed diets, weight gain, and almost suicidal despair she went on a crash diet and told her doctor that the weight loss was due to having become bulimic. She has now been referred to the clinic for eating disorders which would not take her when she was wrestling with the pain of being outcast and fat. She says she has never vomited or used laxatives but deliberately lied her way into the clinic. She is now receiving psychotherapy which is helping her confront her problems with eating and weight. She says she feels that she is being listened to for the first time — her non-existent bulimia has made her acceptable. And who can blame her?

Britain has a long way to go. In the United States there is a nationwide organisation called AHELP — The

Association for the Health Enrichment of Large Persons. This multidisciplinary professional body is dedicated to: professional exchange that advances acceptance, support and treatment of large people; to research that furthers the understanding of factors which both enhance and undermine the health of large people; to professional and societal acceptance of large people and to professional and societal education about the inappropriateness and dangers of weight–reduction dieting. British medical profession and health–care workers please take note. As David Garner and Susan Wooley say in the concluding paragraph of their report: 'Considering what is currently known about obesity and its treatment, we believe it remarkable that there have been so few calls for the re-examination of the fundamental premises that form basic health care policy regarding weight loss.'

To diet or not to diet? That is no longer the question.

9

Where to from here?

Since I wrote the first edition of this book, five years ago now, I have not dieted. What I have done, following the advice of a nutritionist friend, is to eat a very low-fat diet. This was quite difficult to achieve because I am a vegetarian and already ate very little in the way of fats. However, I cut them down still further and it has become, for me, a pleasant way of eating. I love granary bread and bananas, and whole oats with dried fruit and seeds, pumpkin and sunflower, all covered with plain yogurt. My eating exploded one dietary myth — that if you don't include a lot of fat in your diet you lose weight. I have lost nothing! Somebody else with a different genetic make-up, a different metabolism and a different dieting history may well have lost several stones, a vast number of pounds. It just serves as another illustration of the fact that fat people cannot easily lose weight and do not stuff themselves with the clichéd cream cakes.

This year I have changed my diet slightly as have many people in Britain. I now use lovely, fruity, green extra-virgin olive oil for cooking, for salads, to drizzle onto vegetables or oven-toasted bread covered with tomatoes and herbs. I have been investigating food books (some are listed at the back) and I will not have a book in the house which masquerades as a healthy-eating plan and turns out to be a diet. The one I recommend — with one or two small reservations — is the *Mediterranean Health Diet* by Gilly Smith and Rowena Goldman. The word diet in the title does not mean weight loss. This book is a story, the tale of a search and a journey. A band of doctors, nutritionists and health researchers set out to find where in the Western world they could find a country or an area with the lowest incidence of premature death and illness. They discovered such a community in southern Italy where heart disease and cancer are relatively unknown. Having discovered the place, they investigated the diet and found it high in one ingredient — olive oil. Among this group of seekers was Professor Ancel Keys, now 90, whose work on obesity and the hazards of dieting went unheard for 40 years. He and many of the researchers so loved the place they had discovered, the happy, healthy people and the wonderful food, that they retired there. So has the former Finnish Surgeon General, Martti Karvonen, who had been one of the few to listen to Professor Keys and who saw to it that Finland changed its high-risk diet with its appalling results. This book is full of anecdote, good nutritional information, and stories from all sorts of people connected with food. It's a good read and the Mediterranean recipes are delicious. The reservations I mentioned are that the authors occasionally get slightly censorious about overweight, but these bits are not enough to spoil the book and I just ignored them. I do strongly believe in eating good food and not junk and I consider this book the best basis I have found for a really good eating plan. Who knows, you *may* lose weight without trying even if I'm destined not to do so.

My daughter has a mug with a picture on it of one of her favourite characters, the cartoon cat, Garfield. His expression is desolate as he contemplates a plate with miniscule portions and his thought balloon says: DIET IS DIE WITH A 'T'. We could do a lot worse than take fat, funny Garfield as a role model, with his philosophy of a lasagne-loving, Monday-hating life! He is one of the few, much-loved fat images that society has well and truly taken to its thin-worshipping heart.

It would be no bad thing to remember Garfield's diet slogan. I hope that the overwhelming evidence that being fat is not a sin nor does it damage your health will take the pressure off anyone who constantly feels that she must diet — again. I have only been able to show you the tip of the iceberg of the medical evidence; there are hundreds of books, and studies and scientific papers, a massive amount of research carried out in different countries, with different age groups, types, women, men, children, using different controls. One of the immoral facts of the pressure to be thin is that we do not have ready access to this information — it is not the kind of thing you find in women's magazines. It took a good deal of research to track it down but having found it, I hope that all fat women will feel reassured by it.

It may be enough to convince you that you really do not need to and should not diet. If I have learnt one thing it is that dieting is the most hazardous thing we do to ourselves; one of the great health risks we take time and again. As fat women I believe we have to make an informed decision, make it once and stick to it.

If you really feel you want to lose weight, either because you cannot bear the social abuse any longer, or if you come into the 'morbidly obese' category, then please think very carefully about how you do it. Don't attempt to lose a great deal of weight; that is unrealistic and you end up feeling defeated. Don't use the Cambridge Diet or any like it, or any fad diet. The ones we have had in the past have all proved to be unsafe — like the Mayo Clinic diet where you stuffed yourself with cholesterol laden eggs all day. The Doctor's Quick Weight Loss Diet is out because it is high protein, low carbohydrate; it would be out anyway, as is any diet claiming quick weight loss. The thing to remember is that people who write diet books do so to make vast amounts of money because one thing that is sure of selling is a diet book. Judy Mazel's book, *The Beverley Hills Diet* was condemned by doctors, nurses, nutritionists and government agencies, but that didn't stop her promoting it on chat shows right across America. The diet relied on eating a lot of fruit and getting diarrhoea. 'If you have loose bowel movements, hooray', she says. One American writer called it the most unpleasant way to lose weight since tapeworms![1]

If you decide to lose weight, please promise yourself that it will be for the last time. Half a pound a week was the amount suggested by a top cardiologist, Celia Oakley. Whatever you do, there should be no 'forbidden' foods — being 'forbidden' by society is more than enough without censoring what we eat!

Cutting out sugar is a good thing — it has no nutritional value, but again, don't deprive yourself. If you have a mainly sugar-free diet, don't yearn for a bar of chocolate and think you can't have it; go and buy one. If you want butter occasionally, have it. A low fat diet should not mean a no fat diet.

If you have, like me, abused your body for years, not by being fat but by alternately dieting and then giving up and filling it with any junk going, it is a good idea to rethink what your body means to you. You may hate it because it is fat, but this is part of the split between body and spirit that occurs in anorexics and fat women. Healing the split is essential whether you decide to lose weight or stay as you are.

You can start by promising yourself that your body is worth feeding properly (even if you don't believe it), and that in order for it to function to its best ability you will only give it good food. Nice food, not 'diet' food. Smoked salmon sandwiches (no, it does not cost a great deal to buy a small piece of smoked salmon very occasionally; you — and I — deserve it). Before you start to think about weight loss, find the right eating pattern and don't think about quantities. Send messages to your body that it will always have enough, that you won't be calling up the starvation/ famine response any more.

If you look back over a lifetime of bizarre eating patterns you will probably be able to isolate moments when you renounced certain foods for life because they were 'fattening'. I gave up butter when I was fifteen and had not had it until recently; it never occurred to me to put it between my toast and whatever I was putting on top, whether jam or an egg. Then I decided to practise what I was preaching in this book, and I had toast and butter. It was wonderful, I had forgotten how good butter tastes. I shall not go mad and plaster it on everything, but I shall incorporate it into my diet (not my dieting) and enjoy it. The old cliché of all things in moderation applies particularly aptly to eating, I think, but don't be pedantic about the moderation bit! If you want the occasional splurge on food, just as people have spending sprees or a drinking night, then do so.

While writing this book I have become increasingly aware that what I have been advocating applies to me. So what am I going to do? With a track record of many stones lost and many more gained, I have been too scared by what I have discovered about the dangers of diet and regain to risk that treadmill again.

While the charts say I should weigh eight stone (112lb) and my ideal weight is thirteen (180lb), I am not happy or comfortable with my present size. This is because, for reasons I haven't discovered, I put on a great deal of weight after the birth of my third baby, sixteen years ago, and have lost and regained in a series of ever increasing swings until I weigh over sixteen stones (225lb). As I am no longer an idealist and have accepted the idea of compromise with age, I do not yearn for the thirteen stones of my twenties but would settle for about fourteen (195lb). Which is to say that relativity needs to be taken into consideration, and while I was happy to be considered fat, I am not pleased at having entered the category of 'grossly obese'. The stigma is greater, and I am not quite sure at the moment what I am going to do about it.

One thing remains clear, however. If I espouse the Earth Mother image of womanhood then it is perhaps better to be vastly overweight, for I see no beauty for me in a body image of thinness. As long as fat women accept Orbach's bald statement that 'We know that every woman wants to be thin' we will never find our real identities.[2] Part of the fascinating search to find out who we really are, to get to know ourselves, involves coming to terms with the idea of accepting ourselves, forgiving ourselves and loving ourselves. If big women remain stuck with the propagandist notion that every woman wants to be thin, then there will be no chance to explore the reality of the whole spectrum of possibilities.

As for Orbach's assertion that compulsive eating is an individual protest against the inequality of the sexes, I for one have a clear picture of my own eating which bears no relation to that statement as far as I can see. I eat under pressure; I eat when I am upset, or worried in the nagging way that underlies everything you do because it is usually about a problem that appears to defy solution. I do not eat when I am relaxed, or when I am being 'fed' by non-food alternatives. An evening with friends, a stimulating lunch date with a colleague, talking, laughing, enjoying another person, puts food in its proper place for me. I believe that every woman's reason for being fat, whether she under-stands it or not, is her own, related to her own personality and personal circumstances.

Whether or not we decide to try to reduce our size, we are still going to be fat women in the eyes of society. The prejudice is not going to go away in the foreseeable future.

We need to find ways to meet this viciousness, and it seems to me that we are once again dealing with the metaphor of meeting the monster, turning and facing the ferocious dog snapping at our heels.

POSITIVE OR PORNOGRAPHIC?

On the other hand, I believe we have to be vigilant, to watch for signs that the anti-diet movement does not take us in the wrong direction. With this particular trend, there are so many bandwagons rolling that the highways are positively jammed with them, so radical is the message that Dieting Is Out. I have said in this book that I admire and identify with positive images of fat women, with the beauty, generosity, abundance and fecund femaleness that these images suggest. Great care was taken over the choosing of the cover of the book because the fat woman's body is an area of extreme sensitivity. I have shown that the majority of fat women feel that they cannot reveal their bodies to anyone else, some not even to a lover, and many cannot bear to look in a mirror. The fat body is essentially a hidden body. Where it *is* displayed — if a large woman goes swimming for instance — you will always find people of both sexes and all ages staring, with disgust, contempt or very often with a voyeuristic fascination. There are vile pornographic magazines which feature fat women; one I saw was the best-selling porno magazine in Germany and showed *only* fat women, some of them performing acts which only a fat woman could do. I was glad I could not understand the text.

Here I find myself in a dilemma. While I long to see positive media images of large women I strongly feel that a fine line must be trodden between salacious, prurient gawping at abundant flesh and strong, honest representation of it. I know I have complained about magazines featuring Big is Beautiful articles in which they show women who are *not* fat but I think we need to be wary of the other extreme. For instance, the July 1993 issue of *Options* featured Jenny Freeman, attractive, successful, married, happy — and fat. Twenty stones (280lb) and with the confidence and self-worth to accept that she was beautiful as she was, she did not need to diet for any reason or for anyone. Her size was no problem to her and she was an inspiration for those who are not able to feel so positive. But she was featured *nude* and I have to ask why. Not surprisingly, she was asked to pose nude for *The Sun*, the most popular British tabloid. In August she appeared in the weekly magazine *Woman*, once again emphasizing her positive feelings about her size but this time fully clothed — in fact, modelling several outfits. Jenny Freeman says she was quite happy to pose nude but did she, I wonder, question the motives behind the requests for her to do so? It can appear so innocent, cloaked under the guise of She's Fat and She's Beautiful and She's Not Ashamed to Show it. But magazine and newspaper editors are primarily concerned with sales and it has to be said that pictures of a naked 20-stone woman would certainly increase sales. People are fascinated at the idea of seeing lots of excess flesh and I am uncomfortably reminded of the spectacle of the fat lady in the circus. I am also reminded of another occasion when a fat woman was photographed for a magazine — in her case because she found her body so repulsive that only by exposing it to the world in this way did she feel she would be shamed into dieting. She did, and the magazine featured a series of nude photos of her from fat to thinner. These are not what I call positive images and Jenny Freeman's attractiveness and confidence was just as evident in the clothed *Woman* article as in the nude ones. I suppose, though, it wasn't as fascinating for the gawpers.

Jenny Freeman says she enjoys going to Planet Big Girl,

a London nightclub for those women who want to dance in an atmosphere where they need not feel self-conscious. The idea in principle is good, given what we know about the pain and embarrassment of being stared at when we try and do 'normal' things (see Chapter 2 — I think there should be health spas where large women can go, too). But Planet Big Girl is run by a woman who calls herself Creamy Clare (cream éclair) who wears tight black leather encaging her 20 stones — and here I must be clear — it is not that I think fat women should not wear these kinds of clothes, it is the pornographic image that goes with them I don't like. She looks like a dominatrix and indeed says that if anyone makes a fat woman feel bad 'they'll be squashed by 10 big girls and force-fed chocolate until they're sorry'.[3] A male customer at the club says he likes big women because he likes to be engulfed; it reminds him of Fay Wray and King Kong.

I am sure I will be accused of prudery and censorship, and that it will be pointed out that one of the things that fat women are fighting for is the right to behave just as thin women always have. But this does not mean I would find the images I have described any more acceptable if the women *were* thin. I am concerned about negative stereotypes of fat women being reinforced (force-fed chocolate, for example) and I am very worried about the pornographic exploitation of fat women. When I look at the photos of a naked fat woman in the tabloid newspaper I cannot help thinking of the German porno magazine; and when I see Creamy Clare in her black leather and read about people being squashed by '10 big girls', I am reminded of the awful Roly Poly Kissogram girls who will sit on a man's lap and engulf him with almost-naked flesh.

MEETING THE MONSTER — A PERSPECTIVE ON DEALING WITH OPPRESSION

Having rejected the blatant depictions of fat women I have just described, I feel that I want to finish on a positive, assertive and optimistic note. I do not believe that we have to make startling statements by posing in the nude or emphasising our right to eat chocolate. I feel that these things will only serve to further alienate our oppressors and will do nothing to reverse the negative stereotyping that society uses as a weapon against us. What we have to do is to turn and meet this oppression, with the certain knowledge that there is *nothing wrong* with being fat. I am not suggesting that we adopt the too-easy solution of immediately feeling good about ourselves — we cannot call that up to order. It will come to us, though, if we devise means of holding onto our self-respect when it is threatened by others, by turning and questioning their motives. I am talking about those in authority, like doctors, and those who hand out gratuitous insults, as well as the spectrum in between. Thinking about this as I walked through London one day made me realize that if I were to put this into practice, then if a workman on a scaffold hurled me a 'fat cow' type of insult I could no longer pretend I had not heard, and walk on burning with anger and humiliation. I would have to challenge him. And the thought terrified me. Workmen were silent that day but on the way home I stopped at a motorway service station for a meal. A group of five men sat at a table just far enough away for me not to be able to hear what they were saying, though from their glances in my direction and their roars of laughter I could guess. When I had finished I walked past them to the exit and caught the mocking laughter and the words 'Cor! What a size'. Heart thumping, I turned and faced them. They looked uncomfortable. I walked up to their table and said

'Is there anything you would like to say to my face, rather than behind my back?' They mumbled something that might have been an insult, a defence or an apology — I couldn't tell. I walked away, this time without being followed by jeers or laughter. A small victory and one that cost me a lot, but next time I will be much bolder.

We owe it to ourselves to do this, and we owe it to the people who are perpetrating this persecution. It will make them think, even though they will probably bluff it out. Most people, though, are not entirely without shame or conscience; in this sort of thing they act very often out of ignorance, habit and a long tradition of baiting the old, the fat, the disabled. Their insults might be half-hearted next time a fat woman walks by and eventually they will stop, like the bully in the playground who only draws power from the fear of those who appear to be weaker.

The pain of being outcast and vilified does not mean that we must wait helplessly for the world to accept us as we are. Fat is not a feminist issue, it is a political and a humanist issue. It is very easy to feel alone and to give way under the onslaught of hatred, especially if you are the only one in your immediate circle who is fat — but we must *not* allow our oppressors to go on winning. While we long for acceptance, the reality is that true fat acceptance may not come in our lifetimes but that fact in no way diminishes the truth.

Vivian Mayer, a wonderful fat activist who started a Fat Liberation movement in the early 1970s in California, had a tremendous struggle to make the collective voice of oppressed fat women heard. She and others compiled an anthology of fat women's writings — *Shadow on a Tightrope* — but they could not get it published. Even left-wing presses reacted unfavourably to the manuscript — 'They could not believe that fat could be other than a sickening condition caused by bad eating habits.' And while feminist presses were more open-minded to the idea, they too turned it down but felt the book would appeal to a small minority only — women who 'liked' to be fat. So Vivian Mayer distributed the book herself. The fact that it is available now shows that there has been some movement in the United States in the last 20 years.

We cannot sit back and wait for the world to change and accept us — we *must* find the courage and integrity to challenge everyone who puts us down, or suggests that we would be 'better' if we were thinner. If you need to whip up a bit of anger to give you this courage, just think about the fact that fatness is the only aspect of physical appearance that people seem to feel they can comment on without the usual social restraints. People who say 'Have you always been big? Have you ever tried to lose weight?' would never, in normal social interaction, make remarks such as 'Have you always had a problem with acne (or greasy hair or crooked teeth?) Have you thought of going to see an orthodontist?'

There are times when it seems hopeless, when you feel beaten by the enormous power of the persecution, especially if you are feeling low, unwell or depressed. It can be all too easy to internalise the hurt and this is something we must watch out for. If we let things pass they will damage us, the pain will fester and add to the accumulation of layers which we have been building over the years. The result is more stress and a sense of disempowerment. Anger — what religion calls 'righteous anger' — is what we need but we also have to forgive ourselves for the times we let 'them' get away with it. We are not omnipotent and most of us are so sensitised to this hatred that it can be like a raw, exposed wound.

Today is Monday. On Friday I had been to see my closest friend, dying of cancer in a hospice. I was saying goodbye to her and I was feeling very vulnerable. On Saturday I was browsing around the town with a friend and stood in a small courtyard of shops, waiting for her to finish paying for her purchases. It was warm and sunny, there were chairs and tables there with people eating and drinking and I stood meditating for a few moments, thinking about my dying friend. A small child, about four years old, walked past me with her mother. 'Look' she shouted, pulling at her mother's arm. 'Look at that fat lady. *Look* — there!' — urgently, lest her mother should miss this terrible sight. I felt humiliated, naked, exposed, helpless. I was rooted to the spot. I did and said nothing. On Sunday a friend who was visiting me commented on a photo of me with my baby — taken when I was 28 and weighed quite a lot less than I do now. 'You looked wonderful — *then*' she said. I didn't challenge her. On Sunday evening another woman moaned to me about her weight. 'But you are not overweight by *any* standard' I told her. 'No you're right' she agreed. 'But if I lost weight, I could get rid of *this*' indicating her hips and bottom. I told her of the research about the protective factor of the 'pear shape'. She has high blood pressure and a family history of strokes and heart attacks. But the dreaded hips obviously caused her more concern than what I had said. At last I got angry. 'Hearing things like that makes me think *what is the use of writing this bloody book*' I shouted. It was the right reaction. She was startled and this made her think. Then, only then, was she ready to hear what I had to say.

Today I heard that my dying friend has slipped into unconsciousness. She was a fat woman who had been healthy all her life. Nothing laid her low until the cancer, and it was not the type that large women are susceptible to. I sat thinking about her, remembering the last time I saw her out of bed, a few weeks ago. She had lost seven stones, her skin hung in folds. 'I may have wanted to lose weight at times' she said. 'But not like this. Never like this.' For me, that puts everything into its correct perspective. Those who hate and fear fat, who have to harass and persecute those of us who are fat, those who are average size and who are constantly preoccupied with losing weight — this poses deep questions about the real meaning of life's priorities and about the relationships between all human beings. About what is *really* important. But there will be no overnight revolution and so it is important that we keep working for change, to develop the habit of non-acceptance where fat-baiting is concerned. To forgive ourselves and make allowances for the times when we miss opportunities to confront prejudice, as I did this weekend, remembering that we cannot always be strong activists, that sometimes our own vulnerability will cause us to retreat temporarily. But we must hold in front of us the central ethic of what this is all about. Fat-hatred is the last bastion. We cannot, we *must* not let them continue to get away with it.

Insults in the streets are the crudest form of persecution, but the censuring doctor or employer is no less culpable for having the polish and sophistication of education and profession. It is important that we understand that they are the poorer for their lack of understanding. People's belief systems, especially those of medical professionals, are based on the fat is bad ethic and that is going to take some power to shift. We need patience and perseverance, and the knowledge that whatever we think about ourselves it is a *fact* that our worth does not depend on our weight. We should be aware of all the tricks of the treacherous compensating personality, and not collude with it. We do not need to apologise for existing.

I was entering a shop that had rather a narrow doorway and a customer waiting to come out said, "If you get any fatter you won't be able to get through that door." I replied: "Perhaps not, but fortunately my size doesn't seem to affect my manners."

> I was walking through the bar of a pub which was rather crowded. I brushed past a woman as I squeezed through and heard her mutter "fat cow" or something like that. I turned round and said sweetly, "Isn't it a good thing *you* don't have to rely on your personality!"

I feel that a ready, witty riposte, or a serious challenging of people's insensitivity is the most powerful and effective way to make ourselves heard. If we return the abuse we are not only colluding with the perpetrators, we are fuelling the fires of those who would believe that fat means unstable, out of control.

We in Britain can learn a lot from NAAFA who have an impressive track record of getting things done. It does not depend on the fact that it is a large organisation with an impressive advisory board — its members have achieved a great deal from individual actions. Letter-writing is more effective than you might think — people are not used to being challenged. Write to anyone, company or individual, television programme or magazine, who does or says anything offensive. Remember that they could not do it to black or disabled people. We and the elderly are the targets now but it is surprising how sensitive the most unlikely people can be. We do not have to be victims and the best way of getting out from under the victim state is to take action. I recently wrote to a number of women's magazines that had been running an advertisement for a diet product making completely fraudulent claims. The magazines all thanked me for pointing this out and the advertisement was removed. Join Dietbreakers and NAAFA — it does a great deal to put an end to the isolation so often felt by large women.

Write down the things that you hear other people say in their defence and use them. Write letters to any professionals who use your weight as a definition. Query things: I was told I had to have a medical in order to get a joint bank loan with my husband who was not summoned for examination. I telephoned and queried the medical grounds for this, refusing to accept overweight *per se*. It was quite amicable and in the end they said I did not need the medical after all.

And if you can, see the humour in the situation, somewhere, even if it is only a glimmer. I have never liked 'fat' humour, entertainers using their fat to make people laugh at them. I find it too sad, the tears of the clown again. But I saw a fat woman wearing a badge which made me laugh out loud and I still chuckle when I remember it. It said: 'Gain Weight Now: Ask Me How'. You may not see anything funny in that — humour is an individual thing, but somehow in this bleak situation, it is there for all of us.

Don't let your friends make sympathetic or would-be helpful suggestions. What they are saying is, 'You are not acceptable as you are now'. Tell them that their remarks are hurtful or that you find them in bad taste. You won't lose any *real* friends, but you will give them an awareness and sensitivity that they did not have because of their ignorance, because we keep making it alright for them to say these things. All part of the compensating personality again.

I started this book with a letter, a sad letter that made me angry on its writer's behalf. I would like to end it with a quite different letter:

'I am 21 and I weigh 18 stone, the eldest of seven children. I work every evening in a petrol station as a cashier — not the world's most thrilling job, but never mind! My ambitions are to be a writer or a singer — maybe both.

Now down to the nitty-gritty. I've been fat since I was 14 and been on countless unsuccessful and uninspiring diets. Each time it has been because other people have badgered me into losing weight. To be honest, I'm perfectly happy the way I am and I have no intention of changing just because someone else thinks I ought to weigh less. My mother is always on at me to lose weight and I feel like screaming: LEAVE ME ALONE!!! THIS IS MY BODY AND I'M STAYING THIS SHAPE BECAUSE THIS IS THE WAY I FEEL COMFORTABLE.

When I was at school I was picked on and called names but it didn't upset me too much — I realized that children will always find something to tease you about.

What really riles me is folk who say things like "How long have you had your weight problem?" I just smile (through gritted teeth!) and say "It's the way I am and if you think there's something wrong with me, it's you who have got the problem".

I don't judge others by their appearance and would expect them not to do so either, but unfortunately it doesn't always work out that way. I just want to be accepted as I am — a normal, everyday person who just happens to be bigger than average. If people are shallow enough to judge me by looks alone, then they're not worth bothering about.

I've always said, about my size, THOSE THAT MIND DON'T MATTER AND THOSE THAT MATTER DON'T MIND.'

I do not know how a young woman of twenty-one, whose mother does not accept her fat, manages to have such a happy and balanced outlook. I feel that she must be a very special person. She has learnt to live happily in a hostile world and so she is likely to meet less hostility than most people. She cannot tell us *how* to do it but any fat woman who feels unhappy about her body, her shape, her size, her self, could surely do no better than to take, as a sort of mantra, that last epigrammatic phrase of this letter, and say it over and over again to herself until belief in the truth of those words starts to break through the anger of the unfriendly world.

Further reading

Where I have given a British or American publisher, it is likely that the books can be obtained on the other side of the Atlantic as well.

Armstrong, Karen, *The Gospel According to Woman – Christianity's Creation of the Sex War in the West,* London, Elm Tree Books/Hamish Hamilton Ltd., 1986

Bell, Rudolph M., *Holy Anorexia*, Chicago and London, University of Chicago Press, 1985

Bennet, William and Gurin, Joel, *The Dieter's Dilemma,* New York, Basic Books, 1982

Brown, Laura S. and Rothblum, Esther D. (eds.), *Overcoming Fear of Fat,* New York and London, Harrington Park Press, 1989

Bruch, Hilde, *Eating Disorders: Obesity, Anorexia Nervosa and the Person Within*, London, Routledge and Kegan Paul, 1974

Bruch, Hilde, *The Golden Cage: The Enigma of Anorexia Nervosa,* London, Open Books Publications Ltd., 1978

Cannon, G. and Einzig, H., *Dieting Makes You Fat*, London, Sphere, 1983

Charlton, Belinda, *Big Is Invisible*, London, Robin Clark Ltd., 1985

Chernin, Kim, *Womansize – The Tyranny of Slenderness,* London, The Women's Press, 1981, New York, Harper and Row, 1981 (under the title *The Obsession*)

Chernin, Kim, *The Hungry Self,* London, Virago, 1986, New York, Times Books, 1985

Cline, Sally, *Just Desserts: Women and Food,* London, Andre Deutsch, 1990

Dyson, Sue, *A Weight off Your Mind – how to stop worrying about your body size,* London, Sheldon Press, 1991

Ernsberger, P. and Haskew, P., *Rethinking Obesity – An alternative View of its Health Implications,* New York, Human Sciences Press Inc, 1987

Greaves, Margaret, *Big and Beautiful – Challenging the Myths and Celebrating Our Size,* London, Grafton, 1990

Greer, Germaine, *Sex and Destiny,* London, Picador

Hall, Nor, *The Moon and the Virgin: A Voyage Towards Self-Discovery and Healing,* London, The Women's Press Ltd., 1980, New York, Harper and Row, 1980

Hirschmann, Jane R. and Munter, Carol H., *Overcoming Overeating,* New York, Fawcett Columbine, 1988

Lewis, C.S., *Till We Have Faces,* London, Fount Paperbacks (Collins) 1956, 1978

Liggett, Arline and John, *The Tyranny of Beauty,* London, Gollancz, 1982

Lorenz, Konrad, *The Waning Of Humaneness,* London, Unwin Hyman, 1988

Louderback, Llewellyn, *Fat Power, Whatever You Weigh is Right,* New York, Hawthorn Press Inc., 1970 (available from NAAFA)

Marwick, A., *Beauty in History,* London, Thames and Hudson, 1988

Morton, Andrew, *Diana, Her True Story,* London, Michael O'Mara, 1992

Mulvagh, Jane, *The Vogue History of Twentieth Century Fashion,* London, Viking, 1988

Myskow, N. with Grose, R., *Love, Sex and the Pursuit of Chocolate,* London, Angus and Robertson, 1990

Ogden, Jane, *Fat Chance: The Myth of Dieting Exposed,* London, Routledge, 1992

Omichinski, Linda, *You Count, Calories Don't,* Manitoba, Hyperion Press, 1992 (available in Britain from Dietbreakers, see Useful Information)

Orbach, S., *Fat Is a Feminist Issue: How to Lose Weight Permanently Without Dieting,* London, Hamlyn Paperbacks, 1979

Palmer, Gabrielle, *The Politics of Breastfeeding,* London, Pandora Press, 1988 and 1993

Polivy, Janet and Herman, Peter, *Breaking the Diet Habit,* New York, Basic Books, 1983

Pollack Seid, Roberta, *Never Too Thin – Why Women are at War with Their Bodies,* New York, London, Prentice Hall Press, 1988

Redgrave, Lynn, *Diet For Life,* London, Michael Joseph, 1992, (U.S.A., Dutton, 1991)

Roberts, Nancy, *Breaking all the Rules,* London, New York, Viking Penguin, 1985

Rowe, Dorothy, *Beyond Fear,* London, Fontana, 1987

Schoenfielder, Lisa and Wieser, Barb (eds.), *Shadow on a Tightrope – Writings by Women on Fat Oppression,* San Francisco, Aunt Lute Book Company, 1983 (available in Britain from the Fat Women's Group, see Useful Information)

Schwartz, Hillel, *Never Satisfied: a Cultural History of Diets, Fantasies and Fat,* New York, Doubleday, 1986

Scott Beller, Anne, *Fat and Thin – A Natural History of Obesity,* New York, Farrar Strauss Giroux, 1977

Storr, C., *Mrs Circumference,* London, Andre Deutsch, 1989

Stuart, R.B., and Jacobson, B., *Weight, Sex and Marriage,* London, W.W. Norton & Co., 1987

Tolmach Lakoff, Robin and Scherr, Raquel L., *Face Value: The Politics of Beauty,* London, Routledge and Kegan Paul, 1984

Welbourne, Jill and Purgold, Joan, *The Eating Sickness,* Brighton, The Harvester Press Ltd., 1984

Woodman, Marion, *The Owl Was a Baker's Daughter,* Toronto, Inner City Books, 1980

BOOKS ABOUT HEALTHY EATING AND LOVELY FOOD!

Davis, Adelle, *Let's Get Well,* London, Thorsons, 1992 (first published 1966)

Smith, Gilly and Goldman, Rowena, *The Mediterranean Health Diet,* London, Headline, 1993

Spencer, Colin, *The New Vegetarian,* London, Gaia Books, 1992

Till, Antonia (ed.), *Loaves and Wishes – Writers Writing on Food,* London, Virago, 1992

van Straten, Michael and Griggs, Barbara, *Superfoods,* London, Dorling Kindersley, 1990

FICTION

Ashworth, Sherry, *A Matter.of Fat,* London, Signet, 1991

Atwood, Margaret, *The Edible Woman,* London, Virago, 1990

Atwood, Margaret, *Lady Oracle,* London, Virago, 1990

Pacter, Trudi, *Kiss and Tell,* London, Grafton, 1989

Sussman, Susan, *The Dieter,* New York, Simon and Schuster, 1989, London, Headline Publishing Ltd., 1989

Weldon, Fay, *The Life and Loves of a She-Devil,* London, Hodder & Stoughton, 1983

GENERAL

Chaitow, Leon, *The Stress Protection Plan: How to Stay Healthy Under Pressure,* London, Thorsons, 1992

Faller, Frank Richard, *Re-create Yourself: Positive Strategies for Self-Development,* London, Thorsons, 1992

Lyons, Pat and Burgard, Debby, *Great Shape: The First Fitness Guide for Large Women,* Palo Alto, CA, Bull Publishing, 1990

Useful information

ORGANIZATIONS

AHELP (Association for the Health Enrichment of Large
Persons) Joe McEvoy Ph.D
Director
Eating Disorders Program
St. Albans Psychiatric Hospital
Box 3608, Radford
VA 24143
USA
Tel: (800) 368 3468

Dietbreakers
Church Cottage
Barford St Michael
Nr Deddington
Oxon
Tel: (0869) 38498

The only really powerful British anti-diet movement.

HUGS
Linda Omichinski
Healthwise Counselling
Box 53028

1631 St Mary's Road
Winnipeg, Manitoba
Canada R2N 3X2
Tel: (204) 428 3432
Fax: (204) 428 5072

Successful anti-diet programme.

NAAFA (National Association to Advance Fat Acceptance)
PO Box 188620
Sacramento
California 95818
USA
Tel: (916) 558 6880
Fax: (916) 558 6881

A human-rights organization 'dedicated to improving the quality of life for fat people through public education, research, advocacy, and member support'.

VITALITY: Promoting Healthy Weight in Canada
Nutrition Programs Unit
Health Services and Promotion Branch
Health and Welfare Canada
4th Floor, Jeanne Mance Building
Ottawa
Ontario
Canada
Tel: (613) 957 8328
Fax: (613) 990 7097

CONTACT GROUPS

Friends for Health
29 Derwent Road
Scunthorpe
South Humberside DN16 2PA
Tel: (0724) 875260

Provides information, a 24-hour helpline and a regular newsletter.

Plump Partners
8 Sealand Avenue
Holywell
Clywd CH8 7BU
Tel: (0352) 715909

Contact group for large men and women and for those who would like to meet them.

Write Weight
c/o South Tyneside Voluntary Project
Victoria Hall
119 Fowler Street
South Shields
Tyne and Wear NE33 1NU
Tel: (091) 456 7007

A contact group for large women. Produces a quarterly newsletter. Unfortunately, most members are still desperately trying to lose weight so Write Weight needs more subscribers who have got off the dieting treadmill.

MAGAZINES AND PUBLICATIONS

Big, Beautiful Woman
9171 Wilshire Boulevard
Suite 300
Beverley Hills
California 90210
USA
Tel: (213) 858 0323

Glossy fashion and lifestyle magazine.

Dimensions
7247 Capitol Station
Albany
NY 12224
USA

'The lifestyle magazine for men who prefer large, radiant women and the women who want to learn about them.' (This must be on the level as it is advertised in the NAAFA newsletter.)

Fat News — Celebrating Fat Women
The Fat Women's Group
Wesley House
Wild Court
London WC2B 5AU

Political newsletter. Copies of *Shadow on a Tightrope* also available.

Obesity and Health
Circulation Department
Route 2
Box 905
Hettinger
ND 58639—9558
USA

Journal for professionals working in all areas related to weight, eating and health. Compulsory reading for anyone who has the care of fat people's health, physical or psychological.

Pretty Big
Pretty Big Publications
1 The Dale
Wirksworth
Matlock
Derbyshire DE4 4EJ
Tel: (0629) 824949
Fax: (0629) 824773

Style and fashion magazine. Subscription only.

Radiance
PO Box 31703
Oakland
California 94604
USA
Tel: (415) 482 0680

Excellent all-round magazine with much input from NAAFA. A champion of fat people's rights and also a very good read.

YES magazine

High-quality publication for large women with a mixture of fashion and editorial content. YES stands for 'You're Extra Special'. Available in Britain from branches of WH Smith.

GENERAL

Amplestuff
W. Fabrey
1150 E Market Street
Charlottesville
VA 22901
USA

Useful items for the large person. Produces newsletter, *Ample Shopper.*

Federal Trade Commission
Correspondence Branch
6th and Pennsylvania Ave., N.W.
Washington DC 20580
USA

Food and Drug Administration
Consumer Affairs and Information
5600 Fishers Lane, HFC-110
Rockville
MD 20857
USA
Hotline: (800) 238 7332

The United States is aeons ahead of Britain in its monitoring of the diet industry. You can get detailed information about the state of the industry, including a brochure, *The Facts About Weight Loss Products,* by writing to either of the above addresses.

Vendredi Enterprises
PO Box 41
Key NAAFA
Camas Valley
OR 97416
USA

Produces a resource directory giving information and sources for everything large people could possibly want or need. Won the NAAFA Achievement Award in 1993.

Notes

CHAPTER 1   CUT DOWN TO SIZE

1 Personal communication with Professor Cary Cooper, Professor of Organisational Psychology, University of Manchester, 9.3.89; Louderback, L., *Fat Power: Whatever You Weigh is Right*, New York, Hawthorn Books Inc., 1970, pp. 161-8.
2 Belinda Charlton included this anecdote with many others in her book *Big is Invisible*, London, Robin Clark Ltd, 1985. It is not a book about being fat however, but about her gigantic weight loss of twelve stones in order to run in the London Marathon. A good read, nevertheless.

CHAPTER 2   PERSECUTION, DISCRIMINATION AND OTHER EVERYDAY HORRORS

1 Ernsberger, P., 'The discriminating doctor', *Radiance*, California, Summer 1987, p. 53. Address for *Radiance*: PO Box 31703, Oakland, CA 94604, USA.
2 *Daily Mail*, 22 March 1989.
3 *Daily Mail*, 15 April 1992.
4 *She*, July 1991.
5 *Daily Mail*, 10 October 1989.
6 Louderback, L., *Fat Power: Whatever You Weigh is Right*, New York, Hawthorn Books, 1970.

7 Allon, N., 'The Stigma of Overweight in Everyday Life', in *Obesity in Perspective* (ed.) G. A. Bray, 1975, pp. 83–102. Proceedings of the Conference sponsored by the J. E. Fogarty International Centre for Advanced Study in the Health Sciences.

8 Myskow, N., with Roslyn Grose, *Love, Sex and the Pursuit of Chocolate*, London, Angus & Robertson, 1990.

9 Rowe, D., *Beyond Fear*, London, Fontana, 1987.

10 Goodman, N., Richardson, S. A., Dornbusch, S. M., and Hastorf, A. H., 'Variant reactions to physical disabilities', *American Sociological Review* 28, 1963, pp. 429–35.

11 Storr, C., *Mrs Circumference*, London, Andre Deutsch, 1989.

12 Allon, op. cit., p. 85.

13 Tertullian, *On the Veiling of Virgins VII*, in *The Writings*, 3 vols, Edinburgh, 1870.

14 Ibid.

15 Armstrong, K., *The Gospel According to Woman – Christianity's Creation of the Sex War in the West*, London, Elm Tree Books/Hamish Hamilton Ltd, 1986. Karen Armstrong shows very clearly that the putting down of women by men started in the very early centuries AD and that holy men hated and feared women's sexuality. While not specifically addressing the question of fat, this book demonstrates the origins of flesh, and therefore fat phobia.

16 Armstrong, op. cit.

17 Aquinas, Thomas, *Summa Theologica IV*, Part I, as quoted in *The Gospel According to Woman*, op. cit.

18 Armstrong, op. cit.

19 Ibid.

20 Ibid.

21 Ibid.

22 New York, Anchor Books, Doubleday, 1986.

23 Ibid., Charlton, op. cit.

24 Allon, op. cit.

25 Ibid.

26 Bovey, Shelley, *Being Fat is Not a Sin*, London, Pandora, 1989.

27 NAAFA Newsletter, December 1992.

28 Maddox, G. L., and Liederman, V., 'Overweight as a social disability with medical implications', *J. Med. Educ.* 44, 1969, pp. 214-20.

29 Reported in NAAFA Newsletter.

30 In addition to personal interviews, many women wrote and asked for a questionnaire to complete as they found that their feelings about being fat were so overwhelming they needed some form of structure within which to express them. One question in the long questionnaire I devised was: 'If you have ever been pregnant, did medical staff give you a hard time on account of your weight?' A number of women were so emotionally damaged by doctors' and midwives' hostility in the vulnerable state of pregnancy that they could not find the courage to face it again. This is an iniquitous example of appalling medical prejudice.

31 Reported in editorial page by Eleanor Graham, *Extra Special*, April/May 1987, p. 4; telephone interview 8 March 1989; von Buchau, S., 'The enchilada nightmare', *Radiance*, Summer/Fall, 1986, p. 14.

32 Telephone interview with author, 8 March 1989.

33 See note 31, above.

34 Ibid.

CHAPTER 3   DYING TO BE THIN – AND DEVELOPING A FAT PERSONALITY

1 Piercy, M., 'It's a crime to get fat', *Cosmopolitan*, February 1989, p. 8.

2 From the Bible — The Gospel according to St Luke, chapter 15, vv. 3-6, 11-32.

3 Graham, Eleanor, editorial in *Extra Special*, July 1988.

4 Linn, R., *The Last Chance Diet Book*, New York, 1976, quoted in *Womansize* by Kim Chernin, The Women's Press, London, 1983, p. 42.

5 Bruch, H., in Louderback, L., *Fat Power*, New York, Hawthorn, 1970.

6 Personal communication, 9 March 1989; Mackenzie, M., *The Politics of Body Size: Fear of Fat*, Los Angeles, Pacifica Tape Library, 1980.

7 Ibid.

8 Mike Wells, Acme Cards, London, 1980. A shrieking example of the strong link between desire for thinness and an affluent society.

9 Maddox, G., Back, K. W., and Liederman, V. R., 'Overweight as social deviance and disability', Duke University, *Journal of Health and Social Behaviour* 9, 1968, pp. 287-97. This quotes several studies of the link between social class and negative evaluation of fatness; in one such study of black and white women and men, the black men were the least condemning; Ernsberger, P., 'It's all in your genes', *Radiance*, California, Winter 1988, p. 34.

10 Ernsberger, op. cit.; Natalie Allon describes the Pennsylvania Rosetans as 'calm, trusting and peaceful' in her discussion of the relationship between temperament and heart disease; she too points out that with their considerable incidence of overweight there was very little heart disease until they 'joined the rat race in the big cities'. Allon, op. cit., chapter 2.

11 Chernin, K., *The Hungry Self*, London, Virago, 1986, chapter 1, which describes the conflict experienced by this woman when she crossed cultures.

12 Mackenzie, M., 'A new US export — fear of fat',

Radiance, California, Winter 1987; Ernsberger, P., op. cit.

13 Ibid.

14 Dr Jill Welbourne in a personal communication; she and Joan Purgold give striking examples of the pressure to succeed/fear of failure syndrome that can lead to eating disorders in their excellent book *The Eating Sickness*, Brighton, The Harvester Press Ltd, 1984.

15 Gomez, J., 'Anorexia — the Safe Rebellion', *She*, February 1992.

16 Knowles, J., in an interview with Anne Robinson in 'Double lives', *She*, September 1988, p. 152.

17 *Options*, September 1988.

18 Marwick, A., *Beauty in History*, London, Thames & Hudson, 1988, pp. 373 and 375.

19 Palmer, G., *The Politics of Breastfeeding*, London, Pandora Press, 1988, p. 32.

20 Glucksman, M. L. and Hirsch, J., 'The response of obese patients to weight reduction', *Psychosom. med.* 31 January 1989 (inter alia); Bruch, Hilde, MD, *The Golden Cage: The Enigma of Anorexia Nervosa*, London, Open Books Publication Ltd, 1978; *Eating Disorders: Obesity, Anorexia Nervosa and the Person Within*, London, Routledge & Kegan Paul, 1974; Woodman, M., *The Owl Was a Baker's Daughter*, Toronto, Inner City Books, 1980. This strangely titled book is a study in Jungian psychology which explores the relationship between fat women, body size and body image. It is very helpful for gaining insight into why we might be fat and how it affects us psychologically at a deep level.

21 In sensitive contrast, Hattie Jacques quoted in *Who's Who on Television*, London, Independent Television Books Ltd, 1988, p. 216.

CHAPTER 4 FRIENDS, LOVERS AND MOTHERS

1 Greer, G., *Sex and Destiny*, London, Picador, 1985.
2 *Sunday Express*, 4 December 1988.
3 Fount Paperbacks (HarperCollins), 1978, first published 1956.
4 Hodder & Stoughton, London, 1983.
5 Shepherd, R., 'Check your mate', *Weight Watchers*, October/November 1987; Stuart, R. B. and Jacobson, B., *Weight, Sex and Marriage*, W. W. Norton & Co., London, 1987.
6 Stuart and Jacobson, op. cit.
7 Shepherd, op. cit.
8 Ibid.
9 February 1989.
10 Venes *et al*, 'Overweight/Obese Patients: An Overview', *The Practitioner* 226: 1102-9, 1982.
11 *NAAFA Workbook – A Complete Study Guide*, available from NAAFA.
12 Quoted by Eleanor Graham in *Extra Special*, October/November 1987. The experiment was conducted at Loyola University, Chicago. Scheimann, E., and Neimark, P. G., *Sex and the Overweight Woman*, New York, New American Library Inc., 1970.
13 Rubel, J., 'When children hate their bodies', and Davis, D., 'Fat phobia and children, myth and reality', *Radiance*, Fall 1987.
14 Ansfield, Alice, editorial, *Radiance*, Fall 1987.

CHAPTER 5 THE TYRANNY OF FASHION

1 Hamlyn Paperbacks, London, 1979.
2 Bovey, S. C., 'Being fat is not a sin' (the seed from which this book grew), *She*, September 1986, p. 88.

3 Schoenfielder, Lisa and Wieser, Barb (eds.), San Francisco, Aunt Lute, 1983.

4 London, Andre Deutsch, 1990.

5 Personal communication, 9 March 1989.

6 Hall, N., *The Moon and the Virgin*, New York, 1980; Bruch, Hilde, *Eating Disorders*, London, Routledge & Kegan Paul, 1974.

7 Chernin, K., op. cit.

8 Marwick, A., *Beauty in History*, London, Thames & Hudson, 1988.

9 Ananth, J., 'Psychological aspects of obesity', *Child Psychiatry Quarterly*, vol. 15, no. 3, July—September 1982, p. 75.

10 Palmer, G., *The Politics of Breastfeeding*, London, Pandora Press, 1988.

11 Mackenzie, M., 'The pursuit of slenderness and addiction to self-control — an anthropological interpretation of eating disorders', *Nutrition Update*, vol. 2, California, 1985.

12 Macleod, H., 'Fit to bust', *Ms London*, 6 March 1989, p. 14.

13 Morton, Andrew, *Diana, Her True Story*, London, Michael O'Mara, 1992.

14 'A Weight Off Her Mind', *Sunday Express Magazine*, 15 January 1989.

15 Mulvagh, J., *The Vogue History of Twentieth Century Fashion*, London, Viking, 1988; Jane Mulvagh also wrote a very good article on the 'fatal attraction of thinness' called 'Naked truths', *Sunday Times Magazine*, 12 March 1989.

16 Mulvagh, 1989, op. cit.

17 Marwick, A., *Beauty in History*, London, Thames & Hudson, 1988.

18 Roberts, N., *Breaking All the Rules*, Viking, 1985.

19 *The Visitor*, (Somerset regional magazine), March 1989.

20 Mower, S., 'As large as life', *Observer*, 27 September 1987.
21 Hands, N., 'New Sensuality of the Big Girl', *Daily Mail*.
22 Wald, D., 'Generous Measures', *Ms London*, 6 March 1989.
23 Neustatter, A., 'Accentuate the positive', *Country Living*, October 1987.
24 Fabrey, William J., 'Individual Acts Spark Political Change', *Radiance*, Fall 1990.
25 'Big Girls Don't Cry', *Cosmopolitan* (London), January 1993.
26 *Radiance*, Fall 1988.
27 Fowler, Alice, 'I put on ten stone and became invisible', *Daily Mail*, 30 December 1992.
28 Pacter, Trudi, *Kiss and Tell*, London, Grafton, 1989.
29 Reported by Eleanor Graham in her editorial in *Extra Special*, October/November 1987.

CHAPTER 6   YOUR LOSS IS THEIR GAIN — DIETS AND THE DIET INDUSTRY

1 Schwartz, H., *Never Satisfied: A Cultural History of Diets, Fantasy and Fat*, New York, Doubleday, 1986. I am grateful to Hillel Schwartz for providing such accessible information in a wonderful, witty treasure-house of a book.
2 Louderback, L., *Fat Power*, New York, Hawthorn Books, 1970.
3 This figure appears in the majority of articles and discussions about women, fashion and weight and it varies from 50–60 per cent; some claim an even higher percentage when size 14 is brought into the equation. Extensive research has failed to locate the source of this figure so I shall just quote one instance of the many times I came across it. In the first issue of the magazine *Extra Special*, now axed by Maxwell, Eleanor Graham

opened her editorial page with: 'Half the women in Britain need a 16 or larger dress size' (October/ November 1986).

4 'Obesity', a report of the Royal College of Physicians, *Journal of the Royal College of Physicians of London,* vol. 17, no. 1, January 1983.

5 Ibid.

6 Cannon, G., and Einzig, H., *Dieting Makes You Fat,* London, Sphere, 1983.

7 London, Pan Books, 1986.

8 The *Independent* newspaper featured Katahn's Rotation Diet on its health page for four consecutive weeks from 19 April–10 May 1988. Health correspondent Oliver Gillie pronounced it Diet of the Decade for reasons I am unaware of and which puzzle me as it is not intrinsically sound dietarily.

9 15 December 1992.

10 Keys, A. *et al, The Biology of Human Starvation,* University of Minnesota Press, 1950.

11 Louderback, L., op.cit.

12 Knowles, A., 'The food of love', *Extra Special,* October/ November 1987, p. 7.

13 Price, J., 'Food Fixations and Body Biases', *Radiance,* Summer 1989.

14 Virago, London, 1986, pp: 177–81.

15 Redgrave, L., *Diet for Life,* London, Michael Joseph, 1992. First published in the US by Dutton in 1991.

16 NAAFA Newsletter, March 1990.

17 Bovey, S.C., *She,* September 1986, p. 88.

18 Ibid.

19 Study quoted by Dr Paul Ernsberger and Dr Paul Haskew in *Rethinking Obesity – An Alternative View of its Health Implications,* New York, Human Sciences Press Inc., 1987.

20 *The Use of Very Low Calorie Diets in Obesity,* DSS (from HMSO).

21 Shepherd, Rose, 'Liquid Assets', *Sunday Times* (London), 21 October 1990.

22 *You* magazine, 25 January 1993.

23 *Dispatches,* Channel Four, 15 December 1992.

24 Bernice Weston talked to Alexandra Campbell in 'Double lives', *She,* January 1989, p. 120.

25 Dr Andrew Hill, Leeds University, England.

26 15 December 1992.

27 NAAFA Newsletter, July 1991.

28 On the day of Christina Onassis' funeral in October 1988, when speculation that her death had been caused by slimming pills was rife, women appeared on 'Kilroy' talking about the destructive and life-changing effects of these pills.

29 Ferriman, A., and Merritt, J., 'Scandal of the slimming clinics', *Observer,* 13 March 1988.

30 Thomas, D., 'I Have ways of making you healthy', *You* magazine, *Mail on Sunday,* 10 January 1993.

31 *Company,* June 1985.

32 Jackson, S., 'Fat suction — trying it for thighs', *Vogue,* October 1988.

33 Medical Advisory Service, 10 Barley Mow Passage, London, W4; Harley Street Medical Advisory Service, 071-935 0619.

34 Woodman, S., 'What it means to be big in America', *Independent,* 4 October 1988; Ernsberger, P., 'The unkindest cut of all — the dangers of weight loss surgery', *Radiance,* Summer 1988, p. 44.

35 Ibid.

36 Purves, Libby, 'Surgery, A Slimmer's Last Resort?', *Radio Times,* 14 March 1992.

37 *40 Minutes,* BBC TV, 17 March 1992.

38 Woodman, op. cit., Ernsberger, op. cit.

39 Ibid.

CHAPTER 7 SO YOU THINK YOU'RE FAT — THE HEALTH FACTS AND FIGURES

1 Quoted in 'Obesity', a Report of the Royal College of Physicians, 1983.
2 Ibid.
3 Ernsberger, P., 'Hazards of drastic loss and regain', *Physician and Patient*, 1985, USA; Ernsberger, P., and Haskew, P., *Rethinking Obesity*, Human Sciences Press Inc., 1987, details several studies on the adverse effects of dieting.
4 Ibid.
5 Personal communication; op. cit. note 9.
6 Andres, R., 'Effect of Obesity on total mortality', *Int. J. Obesity* 4, 1980, pp. 380-6.
7 Waaler, H. T., 'Height, weight and mortality: the Norwegian experience', *Acta Med. Scand.* Supp. 679, 1-56, 1984; Andres, op. cit.; Keys, A., 'Seven countries: a multivariate analysis of coronary heart disease and death', Harvard, Cambridge, Mass., 1980; Ernsberger, P., 'Is it unhealthy to be fat?' *Radiance,* Winter 1986, p. 12.
8 Ibid.
9 Ibid.
10 Ernsberger, P., 'The discriminating doctor', *Radiance,* Fall 1988, p. 53.
11 Ibid.
12 Heart Information Series Pamphlets: no. 11 — 'Reducing the risk of a heart attack', no. 16 — 'Hyperlipidaemia and familial hypercholesterolaemia', no. 7 — 'Diet and your heart'. This is the one where the scientific, objective doctor takes off in flights of emotive and prejudiced prose.
13 'A–Z of positive health', *You,* 5-26 March 1989.
14 Cherreson, A. M., 'The rite to smoke', *Company,* January 1989, p. 56.

15 Chernin, K., *Womansize*, London, The Women's Press, 1983, pp. 33-34.
16 Dr Jill Welbourne provided me with several case histories and much common sense, for which I am indebted to her; statistic from her book *The Eating Sickness*, co-authored with Joan Purgold, Brighton, Harvester Press Ltd, 1984.
17 Ibid.
18 Law, J., 'Pulling your weight', *Weight Watchers*, October/November 1987, pp. 50, 51.

CHAPTER 8   TO DIET OR NOT TO DIET?

1 *Obesity and Health,* September/October 1992.
2 Louderback, L., *Fat Power,* New York, Hawthorn Books, 1970.
3 Ibid.
4 *The Lancet* (UK), 3 May 1969.
5 Materials for this programme are available from Cocono Wellness, 600 N. Dairy Ashford, Box 2197, Houston, TX 77252.
6 Garner, D. M. and Wooley, S. C., 'Confronting the Failure of Behavioural and Dietary Treatments for Obesity', *Clinical Psychology Review,* Vol. II, 1991.
7 Louderback, L., op. cit.
8 Dodd, C., 'Compulsive Eaters Come Out of the Closet', *Independent on Sunday,* 11 July 1993.

CHAPTER 9   WHERE TO FROM HERE?

1 Ben Goelle, J., 'Burn the diet books', *Radiance,* California, Spring 1987, pp. 35, 37.
2 Orbach, Susie, *Fat is a Feminist Issue*, London, Penguin, 1980, pp. 74, 185.
3 Young, Louisa, 'Fat Fights Back', *Marie Claire* (UK), September 1993.

Also published by Pandora

Mothers Who Leave
BEHIND THE MYTH OF WOMEN WITHOUT THEIR CHILDREN

Rosie Jackson

Foreword by Fay Weldon

In Britain an estimated 100,000 women live without their children; in the United States at least half a million. Yet mothers who've left are still thought of as unnatural, deviant, even immoral.

Drawing on her own experience and that of many other women, Rosie Jackson asks what can drive a mother to relinquish her children and examines the emotional aftermath. Exploding the myths that surround such mothers, myths ranging from vampirism to hardhearted feminism, she explores this dark side of mothering with unusual depth and sensitivity.

A close look at popular stories of mothers who leave, from *Anna Karenina* to *Kramer versus Kramer* and *Diana: Her True Story*, contrasts dramatically with the everyday reality of women's actual lives. Alongside a discussion of the most famous examples of such mothers — including Ingrid Bergman, Frieda Lawrence, Yoko Ono and Doris Lessing — Rosie Jackson unearths lesser known ones, introducing some fascinating and moving first-hand accounts.

This is a new, compassionate approach to a controversial and complex subject. Arguing that parenting as we know it must be radically rethought if women are ever to have full and equal lives, Rosie Jackson reveals the shocking personal costs of our double standards and value judgements about mothering.

Trauma and Recovery

FROM DOMESTIC ABUSE TO POLITICAL TERROR

Judith Lewis Herman

'This is a book about restoring connections: between the public and private worlds, between the individual and community, between men and women.' In this landmark study of trauma, the fruit of 20 years of research and clinical work, Judith Lewis Herman, psychiatrist and award-winning author makes the revolutionary link between the 'heroic' suffering of men in war and political struggle and the degraded suffering of women who are victims of rape, incest, and domestic violence. Herman repeatedly challenges established orthodoxies, identifies a new diagnostic category for those suffering from 'hidden' traumas and proposes a ground-breaking recovery programme which favours a process of re-integration to one of catharsis.

A deeply compassionate and readable work, *Trauma and Recovery* is required reading for all those who seek a deeper understanding of the psychology of men and women.

The Tentative Pregnancy
AMNIOCENTESIS AND THE SEXUAL POLITICS OF MOTHERHOOD

Barbara Katz Rothman

As more and more women are having children when they are over thirty, amniocentesis is becoming a routine part of prenatal care. In this groundbreaking book, Barbara Katz Rothman draws on the experience of over 120 women and a wealth of expert testimony to show how this simple procedure can radically alter the way we think about childbirth and parenthood. The results of amniocenteis, and the more recently developed chorion villus sampling, force us to confront agonizing dilemmas very early on: What do you do if there is a 'problem' with the fetus? What kind of support is available if you decide to raise a handicapped child? How can you come to terms with the termination of a wanted pregnancy?

For this new updated edition, Barbara Katz Rothman has written a new introduction and 2 new appendices on the most recent technological advances and the personal and social issues they raise.

Passionate, controversial and at times heartbreaking, *The Tentative Pregnancy* is a must for anyone thinking of having a child and for all those concerned with the growing proliferation of reproductive technology.

Out of Control
MEN, WOMEN AND AGGRESSION
Anne Campbell

In this lucid and highly accessible book, psychologist and criminologist Anne Campbell listens to the voices of men and women as they describe their aggressive feelings, and constructs an intriguing and challenging approach to the vexed topic of gender and aggression. She argues that the crucial difference between female and male aggressiveness is that men see aggression as a means of gaining control over others, while women see it as a loss of self-control. Daughters are deeply ashamed when they get angry, but sons learn to associate aggression with courage and triumph. The implications of this, from rage within intimate relationships and violence in the streets to the attitude of the male establishment — including the judiciary — to women's anger, are searchingly explored.

In an era when women's aggression and the issues of provocation are finally being publicly discussed, Anne Campbells' humane book provides a model of reasoned analysis.